INTELLIGENT

yoga

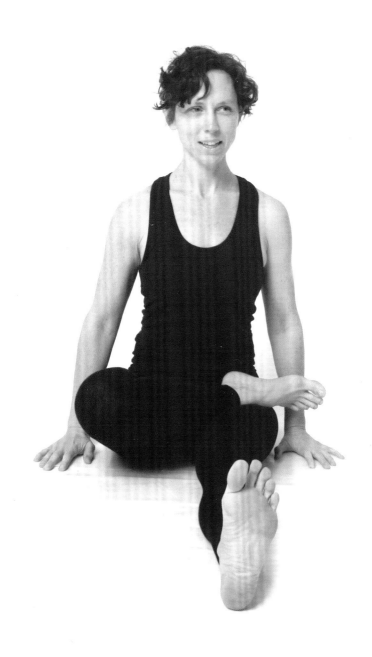

RE-EDUCATING MIND AND BODY

BY PETER BLACKABY

*This book is dedicated to
the memory of my sister
Caroline*

1953 - 2011

First published in the UK by Outhouse Publishing
Copyright © Peter Blackaby and Outhouse
Publishing Ltd 2012

Author
Peter Blackaby

Publisher and Editor
Fiona McWilliam

Art Director
Samuel Blagg

Photographer
Charlotte Macpherson

Illustrator
Nicola Fee

Proofreader
Sarah Thomas

Editorial Assistant
Digby Wheeler

Writing this book has been something of a journey,
and many people have been influential in its
unfolding. I would particularly like to thank the
following for their help in shaping this book: Christine
McHugh, Diane Farrell, Taravajra, Peter Connolly and
Lisa McRory, for their generous sharing of ideas and
practice - I value their friendship; Mary Stewart for her
straightforward and direct teaching; Sarah Thomas
for helping me formulate the beginning and end of
the book; Serge Gracovetsky for his patient answering
of my persistent questions; and Michael Barnes for
introducing me to the wonderful world of yoga.
Finally, thanks to my wife Sabine, and Dominik, my
son, who have had to put up with me when my time
has been consumed by writing.

Photographic sources
All photographs are by Charlotte Macpherson except
for the following: Corbis Images, page 63; Getty Images,
pages 6, 14, 18, 21, 48, 51, 52, 66, 69, 71, 72; istockphoto
(Wingmar), page 22; Press Association, pages 16,
86; Science Photo Library, pages 27, 32, 40, 81; and
Shutterstock (Pan Xunbin), page 31.

The author and publisher have made every effort to
ensure that all the instructions in the book are accurate
and safe, and therefore cannot accept liability for any
resulting injury, damage or loss to persons, however it
may arise.

British Library Cataloguing in Publication Data.
A catalogue record for this book is available from
the British Library.

ISBN-978-0-9572391-0-4 paperback

Printed and bound in Brighton by MCR Print

This book is available from selected good bookshops;
alternatively you can buy it directly from Peter
Blackaby's website www.intelligentyoga.co.uk

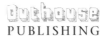

Outhouse
PUBLISHING

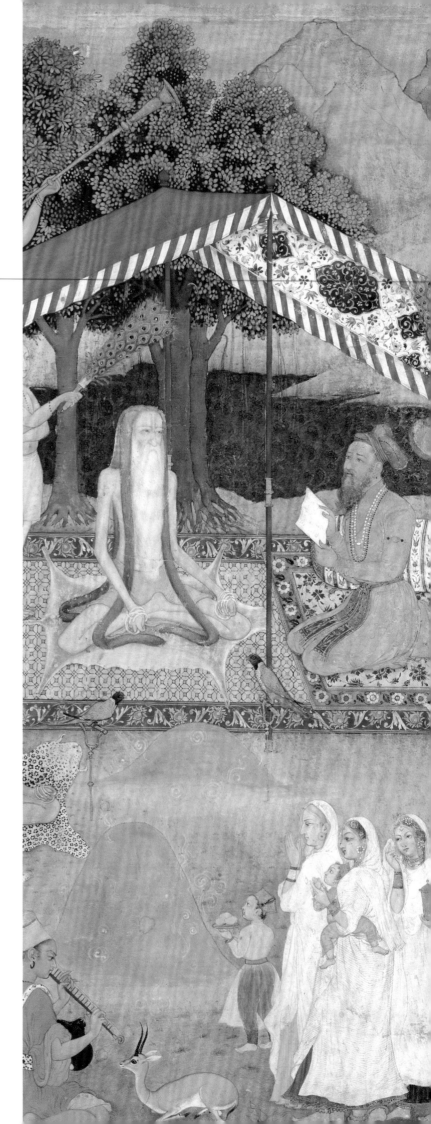

Contents

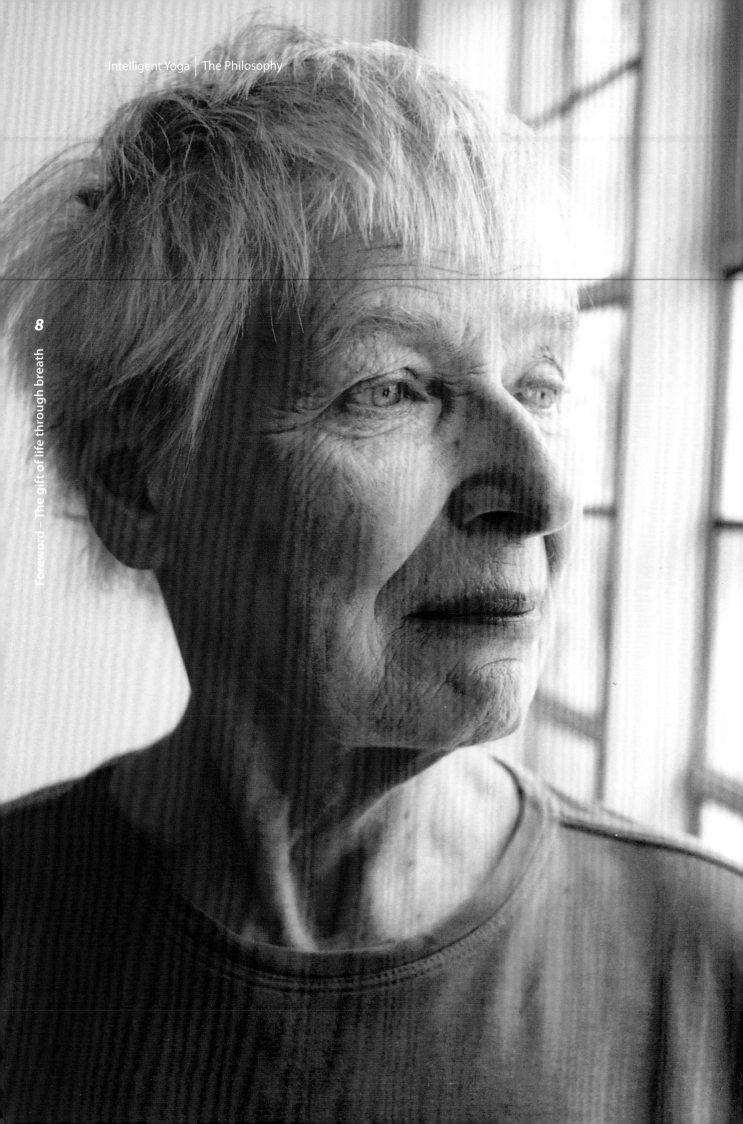

The gift of life through breath

by Mary Stewart

Yoga is India's gift to the world. Pre-dating both Hinduism and Buddhism, it was handed down verbally from teacher to pupil for hundreds of years before it was ever committed to paper.

Most people in the West have heard of yoga, perhaps as a form of keep-fit practised by celebrities, as a weekly class in a local village hall, or even as a dangerous Eastern cult. Yoga has been interpreted in innumerable ways over its long history and there is probably a grain of truth in all its many descriptions.

Yoga as the path to "wholeness" has been taught, elaborated, elucidated, muddled, mystified, hidden and even patented. The huge surge of interest in yoga practice in the West over the past 40 or so years has only added to the confusion, and modern marketing methods continue to spread images of chanting and extreme exercise routines in which the essentials of yoga practice are all too often lost.

The Sanskrit word "yoga" means concentration, but it can also be translated as union. Yoga is additionally defined as "the stilling of the restless state of the mind". The ancient yoga aphorisms of Patanjali advocate an eight-fold path to this end state, the first two steps of which are ethical and moral rules. The third and fourth steps concern bodily posture and the regulation of the breath, and it is these steps, themselves a preparation for the later steps of meditation, which are mostly taught and practised in the West today.

Yoga, being extremely old, has little in common with modern aerobic exercise routines and physical training, despite attempts to market it thus.

"Postures should be steady and relaxed " state the aphorisms; they should be performed by releasing and letting go rather than the through use of effort or force. The postures are a concentration of mind and movement in which the breath undoes the stiffness and tensions of the body, strengthening its weaknesses and restoring health.

As yoga transforms our relationship with our physical selves, our ability to release effort and let go will bring self-knowledge. Doing so is as difficult for the young and flexible as it is for those of us who are older and stiffer.

A sound understanding of our physical selves is essential to those students and teachers wishing to embark on their own yoga journey, and this is what Peter provides here, on the pages of "Intelligent Yoga".

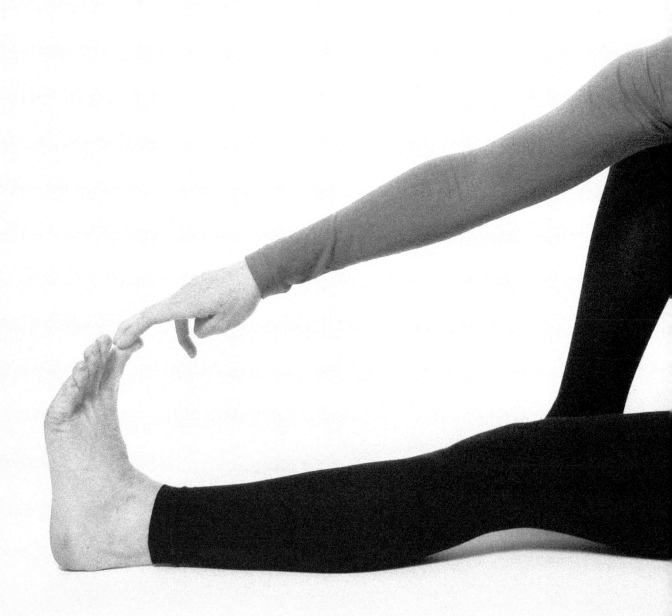

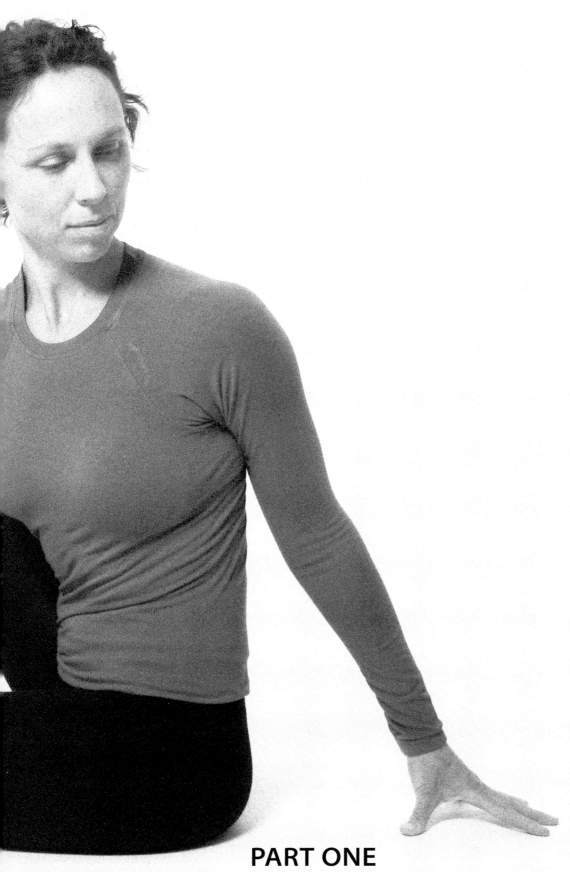

PART ONE

the philosophy

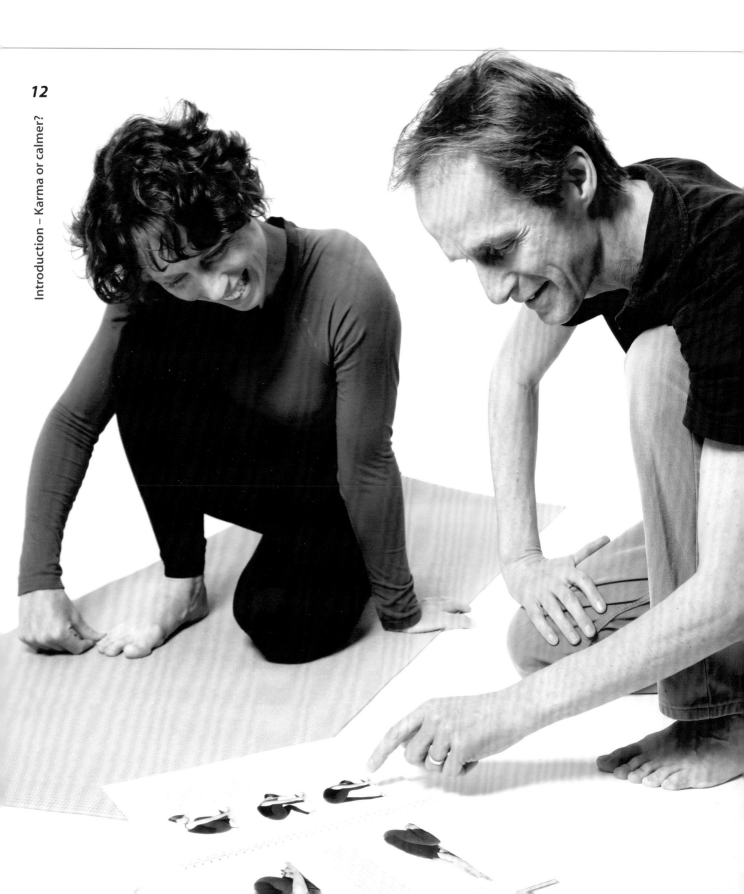

Karma or calmer?

Stories are important; stories provide us with a context for life events. Such events are perceived very differently by different people. For example, a child who chases a ball into the road and is knocked down by a car will have a different set of feelings towards the incident to those of its parents. If the child is very young it may experience the shock and hurt as an unjust and terrifying intervention into an enjoyable game. The parents on the other hand may be wracked by guilt having not paid close enough attention to their child's whereabouts.

Onlookers' responses will vary. Some will be damning of the parents while others, recognising their own fallibility, may show compassion and sympathy. Some may even blame the child. Each will make sense of the event by putting it into the context of his or her own life. Even those who did not witness the event will ask questions about how it happened.

Very few people would be content to hear that a child had been knocked over without wanting to know at least how quickly the car had been travelling or what the child had been doing. In other words, sense needs to be made of events in the light of the experience of the individual.

Yoga, I believe, is no different; it has its own stories and most of us make sense of these stories in the light of our own understandings. We can read, for example, the sacred Hindu text,

the *Bhagavad Gita*. Some will say it is a story about devotion and love, while others will argue that it is a document of social oppression. Some may see both perspectives contained within the same story or may interpret it in a completely different way.

We can choose to take the classic yoga text the *Hatha Yoga Pradipika* either literally or metaphorically. We may read the information about *prana*, *chakras* and "subtle energy", and respond to them with absolute faith, with curiosity, or with complete disbelief.

Within the yoga tradition there are many different stories, each leading us ultimately towards a promised state of "all-knowingness" or enlightenment. Although yoga describes different paths to this goal, somewhere in the heart of yoga is the idea that there is a truth to be discovered – a truth that sees all stories and is not confined by the limitations of the human brain.

It is in this belief that the discipleship found within yoga is rooted. Gurus depend on the belief that they can take us somewhere beyond our own understanding, that they are a necessary conduit for an insight beyond rational thought. Implicit in this view is an historical perspective, a truth was once known by a great teacher or God, and that our aim is to rediscover this truth.

This historical perspective sits quite comfortably within Indian religion, but less so within modern Western thinking, which is essentially forward-looking and explores things

LEFT
We each have our own interpretation of yoga

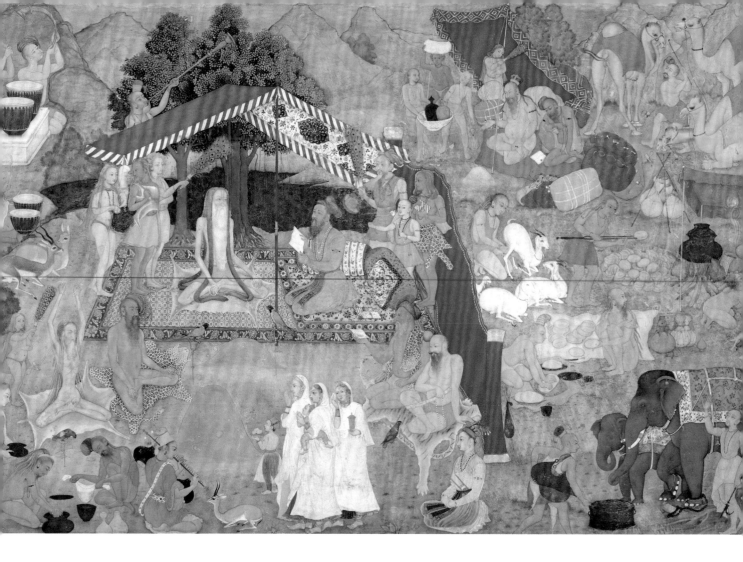

through experimentation, through dialogue and hypothesis.

Of course these are sketchy outlines of two positions that are more blurred in real life, but they nevertheless offer us fundamentally opposing approaches to yoga. It is not helpful to say that one way is right and the other wrong, but I do think it helps if we know in which direction we are facing. The direction I face has changed significantly over the years.

My mother was the daughter of a vicar and had fairly strong Christian beliefs, whereas my father was a science teacher with an evidence-based view of life. As a child I was exposed fairly evenly to both perspectives.

My interest in yoga in my early twenties was driven partly by a need to find answers to life's difficulties, and partly by a desire to find magic. The world I saw at that time (the mid-seventies) seemed fairly grim. Yoga promised a different perspective – in an environment only just emerging from the constraints of post-War thinking.

I dabbled in a few forms of yoga but settled into a regular Iyengar practice. Somewhat to my surprise I found the discipline of this practice

very helpful, as up until then my life had lacked discipline.

For several years, progress in both my life and my yoga were marked. I practised diligently and eventually trained to be a yoga teacher. At this time, I felt a sense of relief in the certainty of the method. To better understand the practice meant simply interpreting the teachings of Iyengar as accurately as possible. There was no encouragement to look at other methods. Rather, one studied with those teachers who had been exposed directly to Iyengar's teaching and, if possible, one learned under Iyengar's direct tutelage.

A certain status was achieved among those students who spent the most time studying directly with Iyengar. I never went to India to study with him, but I attended a few events and classes he led in England. He seemed a frightening but exciting man.

After qualifying as an Iyengar teacher I started training in osteopathy, a career path driven partly by my failing furniture business, but also because it seemed an ideal way of improving my understanding of the bio-mechanics of yoga.

I had started to develop some problems in

The question is whether yoga's success is based entirely on the metaphysical principles expounded in the ancient texts, or whether it can be explained in the light of more recent understandings

my left knee and lower back, and was suffering from migraine headaches. When I presented my physical problems to my senior yoga teachers, they usually suggested that I had missed some nuance in the teaching. Some slight modification to a certain posture would be advised, but this would never be far from the blueprint laid down by Iyengar.

The point here is that the system of yoga I had grown up with was one where the ultimate authority rested with Iyengar himself. I also witnessed his growing status from yoga teacher to that of a guru with a devotional following.

But my osteopathic training and growing anatomical understanding started to reveal discrepancies in what yoga had taught me. This situation was compounded by my meeting John Stirk, a fellow yoga teacher, who was also a lecturer at my college. John's teacher at the time was Mary Stewart. Mary had introduced John to the work of Italian-born yoga teacher Vanda Scaravelli, who had radically reformed the standing postures and developed an approach to posture (*asana*) work that was very different to Iyengar's, despite having trained with him. In retrospect, I realise that this was a significant moment in my life.

What Vanda had shown, and what I was now being exposed to through John and Mary, was that things could change; the authority of the guru was not infallible. I had difficulty digesting this, however, as I had invested a great deal in my Iyengar studies, practice and training. It was now being suggested that there was perhaps another way. Although I did not realise it at the time, this was philosophically a fundamental shift from a backward-looking, historical point of view to a forward-looking perspective.

There is a lot to be said for the historical point of view – a sense of tradition, a certain confidence in the rightness of it all and the camaraderie engendered by shared beliefs. But once doubt creeps in, as it had with my perception of the postures, it becomes difficult not to question what other "certainties" might prove fallible. What about karma and samskara, prana and chakras, kundalini and enlightenment? These concepts loom large in yoga, they are part of its mystery and its attraction; and because yoga is a broad church you tend to find people "inhabiting" different aspects of yoga, preferring one to another. Yet you rarely find one group of yogis saying another group has got it wrong, and that is perhaps part of yoga's charm.

We tend to cherry pick the bits we like and gently ignore the rest. To me, that is a bit like the Bishop of Oxford, saying that he didn't believe in the Virgin Birth, but that his belief in the resurrection was central to his faith.

I feel that this kind of view lacks consistency or discrimination. If you simply pick the bits you like and leave the rest the process becomes arbitrary and, therefore, loses its meaning.

Personally, I have found justifying my belief in yoga to be more complex to resolve than justifying my lack of belief in God. I have no trouble in being "a-theist". I do not believe in God because I see better explanations for the existence of things and no evidence for God's existence.

Yoga on the other hand, when practised intelligently, can help with a host of human afflictions. The question is whether yoga's success is based entirely on the metaphysical principles expounded in the ancient texts, or whether it can be explained in the light of more recent understandings, in a humanist context. This is the starting point for my book.

Pete Blackaby

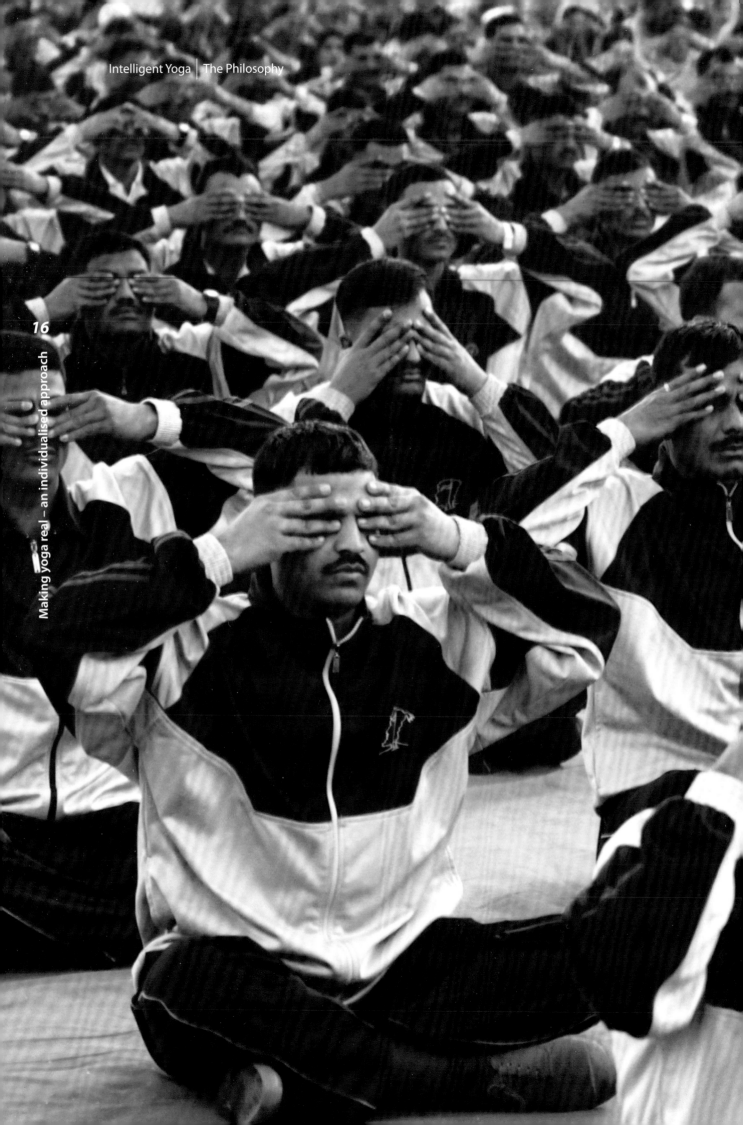

16

Making yoga real – an individualised approach

CHAPTER ONE

Making yoga real: an individualised approach

Yoga is largely an experiential practice and its benefits are sometimes difficult to articulate. Of course it is reasonably easy to explain that an ache or pain has disappeared. More tricky to explain, however, is the feeling of spaciousness in the body, or the clarity of mind that many people associate with yoga practice. These things are harder to express and may necessitate the use of imagery.

We tend to express feelings in metaphors or images in order to help other people interpret our experience. Sometimes this is easy; the feeling of heaviness or lightness for example is something we can all understand. But how does one speak about the transmission of weight through the bones or the subtle changes in tension we feel in our bodies as we breathe?

We cannot even be certain that we are feeling the same thing. If a teacher wishes to convey a sensation as clearly as possible to his or her students then his or her language will by necessity become increasingly elaborate or subtle. This may lead to more complex imagery and, potentially, misinterpretation.

The idea of prana – the Sanskrit word for the vital life-force – could be a case in point. If I am on all fours and I pay attention to my body as I exhale, I can feel a sense of weight or a "release" moving down my arms into the floor. What I am actually feeling is the release of tension that the inhalation necessarily brings into the respiratory system, and the transmission of this

release through the bones of the body and into the floor.

This can be perceived as feeling as if you are breathing out through your arms and exhaling down into the floor. Some people might argue that this is the experience of prana moving down the *nadis* (channels) of the arm as we exhale.

Both descriptions can be helpful to express what is felt and of course different images will work for different people. Problems arise when a description of a "felt sense" is turned into a statement of fact. The statement "it is prana moving down the nadis" brings with it a whole host of assumptions about our physiology, and is quite different to imagining it as a possibility.

Once an idea becomes concrete it is very difficult to open oneself to another experience, as the mind comes to expect what it has been led to believe. Telling someone what they are feeling is quite different to asking someone to take notice of what they feel.

To discuss yoga practice in any meaningful way we should muster as much clarity as possible. It is all too easy to find oneself donning the emperor's new clothes in an effort to comply with a teacher's wishes. If a student is insecure and his or her teacher suggests that a particular sensation or perception is significant, it is likely that the student will say he can feel or see what is suggested whether he can or not. It follows then that if we have a rational explanation for a sensation then we should use it. If we do not, then a neutral image would be better than a

Making yoga real – an individualised approach

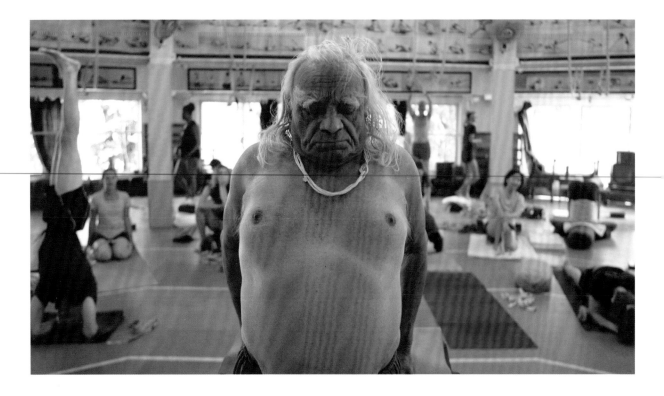

ABOVE
Much of today's yoga practice is based on the teachings of BKS Iyengar

quasi-metaphysical one, or an image that is difficult to "get". This nuance in language may seem a small point but it is the thin edge of a rather large wedge. The more powerfully we assert metaphysical ideas, the less chance we have of allowing people to have their own experience derived from their own practice.

In his ground-breaking early 20th century text *Varieties of Religious Experience*[1], William James suggests that Catholics tend to have Catholic religious experiences, Sufis have Sufi experiences and so on. If a person's experience is to be authentic, it is important that this person is allowed to find his own experience, and discover just how it is for him to inhabit his own body.

Being led to conform to a teacher's personal viewpoint is inevitably disempowering for the student

Being led to conform to a teacher's personal viewpoint is inevitably disempowering for the student, who becomes dependent on the teacher. All power lies with the teacher as the possessor of knowledge. This is the opposite of

what teaching is supposed to do which is surely to facilitate learning as effectively as possible?

A beginner, however, may know nothing of yoga, and so in the early stages yoga teaching has to be directive. Students need to understand how to position their bodies in space, they have to learn the postures in much the same way as a musician needs to learn the fingering of an instrument. Whereas the goal of the musician is eventually to play music, the goal of the yoga student is to feel comfortable in body, breath and mind, and to integrate these aspects of themselves in such a way that there is little or no conflict between them. Once this happens we can start to become truly healthy.

An essential feature of health, which is what we are talking about in its deepest sense, is that we are adaptable and able to rise and respond to changing circumstances, both physically and emotionally. Two observations arise out of this notion. The first is that every individual's experience is unique – it has to be because we are all moulded by our own history. The second observation is that, because we are all human, there are many things that we share. We are unique as individuals but share a common humanity.

Perhaps one of the most challenging aspects of teaching yoga, indeed of life, is the delicate balance between the needs of the individual and the shared human values from which we can all benefit. Students are often encouraged to conform to a particular set of physical and sometimes psychological values. For example, a teacher will provide a sequence of postures to be performed in a particular way and any questioning of this will be met with: "You haven't found the answer because you haven't penetrated the posture deeply enough".

The same can be true when some of the more esoteric ideas in yoga are presented as concrete – the belief that you are not experiencing chakras, auras, or "energy" because you are not yet sensitive enough. The mystery of these things can purportedly be revealed only when you have reached a higher level of understanding.

But what if these things do not exist? Or what if they are phenomena experienced as real by an individual because of his or her personal history? Other people may experience them very differently or may never experience them. If this is the case then any suggestion that these higher states are the result of serious practice can at best only lead to a sense of failure in the student, who doesn't get it; or worse still, it leads students away from their own authentic experience towards a fictitious, supposedly desirable one.

If we change our approach to yoga from one that is systematised to one that is more individualised, we free ourselves from certain constraints. Postures can now be developed around the body, rather than the body around the postures. If a problem occurs with a posture we can look at the posture's biomechanics and try to improve things. This way, should a problem arise – "my knee hurts every time I do this," for example – one can freely adjust the pose so it

is more compatible with one's individual needs.

Solutions to problems in life tend to be sought within the books that are revered by the yogi. In the same way that a Christian might look for solace and answers in the Bible, the yogi might refer to the *Bhagavad Gita*, *Patanjali's Sutras* or the *Upanishads*. Like the Bible, these texts (and others) offer useful insights into ways of reducing suffering but, as with the Bible, they are very much of their time and need serious re-interpretation if they are to make sense nowadays.

How much more sensible it would be to regard them as interesting and valuable historical documents, to which has been added a great deal of perhaps more relevant psychological, philosophical and moral understandings?

If yoga is going to develop in the West, it is necessary to take it forward within the context of the Western mind. Much yogic, and also Buddhist, thinking has at its root the intention of reducing suffering. Life was hard and the tantalising promise of benefits in a future life have long helped ordinary people endure a tough existence.

Life these days, at least for those of us in the West, is different. Although I would be the first to agree that day-to-day living is no cakewalk, there are very few periods of history, if any, I would exchange for the one I live in. We have more choices and freedoms now than at any other time in our civilised past.

While release from harsh physical suffering is no longer the motivation for many people, emotional well-being is something most of us struggle to achieve. Adopting a humanistic approach to living and to yoga, one that is centred around the theme of human flourishing, is the premise underpinning this book.

In the 60s and 70s the West fell in love with

Adopting a humanistic approach to living and to yoga, one that is centred around the theme of human flourishing, is the premise underpinning this book

Making yoga real – an individualised approach

the East, which seemed to offer answers to questions we in the West had not even asked. The ideas of peace, love and understanding that seemed to permeate eastern mysticism sat in stark contrast to post-War scientific thinking, with its much-derided Cartesian, reductive approach to life.

It seemed that Eastern perspectives offered something richer and deeper than the facile lives being lived in the big cities of the West. Of course, we know it is not as simple as that; if the East had so much more to offer than the West, why were countries such as India and China westernising at such a rate?

Pictures of sadhus emerging from McDonald's with whopper-sized milkshakes were not what many of us wanted to see. The West went East and the East went West, and we are still shaking down from the collision of two very different cultures. When these things happen there is an inevitable cross-fertilisation of ideas, some very consciously taken, but others occurring almost by osmosis. It can take a long time before such ideas have sifted enough for sense to be made of them.

Yoga came over to the West as something of a package, and much of what seemed mysterious about it was bound to the culture in which it was embedded. Many thousands of people went to India to experience the authentic setting of yoga. It is unrealistic to expect to import an entire culture and live as an Indian in England or any other Western country, though many tried, and ashrams sprang up all over the Western world.

But things do change and the West has been in the middle of some major transformations over the past 40 to 50 years. Science has led to better understanding of the environment, ecology and the human condition. Thinking

these days is generally less reductionist, so we are starting to better understand the relationship between things. Most people, for example, now realise that not all health problems can be solved by swallowing pills. We know that exercise, diet, stress and environmental factors all play their part in making us healthy or ill.

Initial enthusiasm for the technical fix was scientifically immature. Antibiotics saved millions of lives when they were first introduced, but an over reliance on them has led to problems of microbial resistance. Thinking has had to change, and now it is commonplace to see advice on staying healthy in a doctor's surgery, advice that would have been unheard of even 30 years ago.

Similarly, the use of DDT was very successful in killing mosquitoes and lowering malaria rates, but it was then realised that DDT was also killing much of the wildlife that fed off these insects, so practices changed. Climate change is similarly exercising our thoughts, and many of us are now amending our behaviour in response to what we believe may help mitigate its effects.

Cars today are sold as much for their environmental credentials as they are for their on-road performance, and manufacturers of consumer goods are having to keep pace with the attitudes of a more concerned and informed populace. Thinking is slowly becoming more joined up. Some will argue that there is still a long way to go, but the first steps are being taken.

We have also found flaws in the Indian experience; the Bagwan Rajneesh and his Rolls Royces, and Sai Baba being exposed as a fraudster and possibly worse (even though excuses are still made for him by his devotees). The iniquities of the caste system and the historical support found for it in some of India's

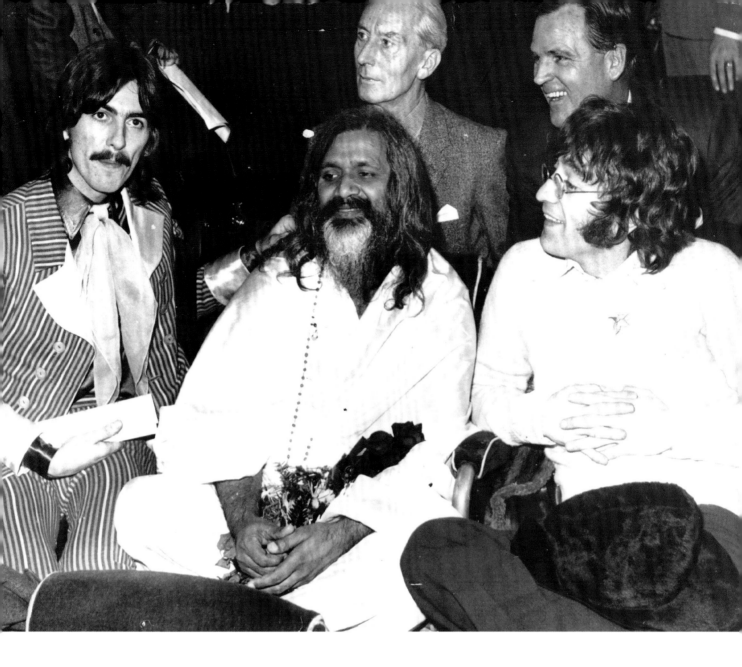

theology and religious texts leave a rather bitter taste in the mouth. It is far too easy to reach ill-informed conclusions about the West or the East, to see these diverse cultures in black and white rather than the many shades of grey that surely exist.

If we start to strip away the culture from yoga and divest it of its metaphysics, what are we left with? And if we do this, can we still call it yoga? These are the questions the rest of this book will explore. I hope to show that there is no loss of dignity in this approach and that in fact there is a great "reasonableness" at the centre of yoga that really works.

There are explanations within the context of the modern Western mind for some of the phenomena that yoga practice brings. The more we are able to use this insight, the greater will be our capacity to adapt and improve what we already have.

For those people who practise yoga on a regular basis there is the undeniable experience that something positive happens. If this book has a purpose, it is to make an attempt at clarifying why this might be.

The benefits that arise from yoga fall into three main categories: benefits to the musculoskeletal system, expressed through a more balanced action of muscles on bones which reduces strain at the joints; an improvement in the responsiveness of the respiratory system, enabling it to meet the needs of changes in effort, emotions and posture; and finally a greater sense of well-being that has something to do with the way we engage with the nervous system, both internally and externally.

It is also apparent that these three facets overlap considerably; improvements in movement tend to improve breathing, improvements in breathing can help movement, and both will have an effect on our sense of well-being.

ABOVE
In the sixties and seventies the West fell in love with the East

22

The fluid body – an anatomy of experience

CHAPTER TWO

The fluid body: an anatomy of experience

To help us understand how we can practise yoga with greater intelligence, it is useful to review the anatomy of the body. But we cannot go back down the old routes of studying anatomy, which is something of a blind alley.

For centuries, anatomy has been investigated by the dissection of cadavers – the study of death. We learn a lot about the position of things by this approach, but we learn little of how the body functions. It is very useful for the surgeon, but for yoga teachers and practitioners this kind of understanding can get in the way.

Most anatomy books still separate out the systems of the body so we can absorb the information in bite-sized chunks. Chapter one might be the skeletal system, chapter two the muscular system, chapter three the respiratory system and so on, with each system seemingly having little to do with the other.

This kind of learning is part of the old reductionism prevalent in much of past Western thinking. If we want to study life and health rather than disease and death we need to make more connections and fewer separations. We need to look at the way the body functions in life and at how the systems interconnect.

Several hundred million years ago evolving creatures crawled out from the oceans on to dry land. These oceans, which had been their home for millions of years, held such importance that they took them with them. Even now, eons after those first land dwellers, we still carry with us the legacy of the sea. Each human being contains about 46 litres of saltwater in the pouches and tubes of their body and the spaces in between. This fluid is constantly pumped, sucked, squeezed and pushed into every conceivable corner of our being. The container for this fluid is the connective tissue of the body, and our health and well-being depends a great deal on the balance and integrity of this tissue.

Overseeing the rhythms of this watery circulation and the integrity of its container is the nervous system, with its distinct autonomic and voluntary branches. In the unborn embryo we see a similar fluid anatomy emerging; the tissues surrounding and separating the fluid contract and expand, forcing pulsations to move through the developing organism. In a watery environment, this pulsation or motility can lead to shape change and small movements. Creatures such as jellyfish use these peristaltic waves of contraction to propel themselves through the water. In the human embryo this pulsation leads to changes of pressure inside the developing chambers of the body, helping it fill out and giving it form.

Shortly after birth, the child learns to organise the anti-gravity muscles that pull her upright, while internally the peristaltic waves of breath and heart continue to impress themselves on the form of the body. The anti-gravity muscles pull us up into standing but they have little to do with holding us there. Instead, together with the supporting bones of the body, the hydraulic and hydrostatic pressures that develop in the chambers of the body create space in the body and resist gravity's compression. Much of the pressure develops in the two large cavities of the body, and is created by the muscles of respiration.

The connective tissue that contains the bodily fluid is given different names in different parts of the body, though its form and function remains basically the same. It is ligament where it joins bone to bone, and tendon where it joins muscle to bone.

There are many more examples of this connective tissue, but all share the function of joining, shaping and containing the human organism. How well it does this depends on the quality of the tissue; in some places it needs to be tough and resilient, in others loose and elastic.

In terms of how this connective tissue organises the human frame we can think of it in two ways. Firstly it is like the guy ropes of a tent, the tensions of the muscles and ligaments pull the skeletal frame this way and that. In a well-balanced frame, these tensions equal each other out so the joints are evenly balanced without stress. In a badly organised structure, joint and spinal problems may develop, or muscular pain and strain.

Secondly, we can think of connective tissue's role in terms of the fluid content of the body. If the connective tissue container supports fluid evenly then pressure will be distributed in a balanced way. This provides hydrostatic support at the core of the human being, taking stress off the spinal column. This support will

allow the spine to lengthen. If the balance of containment is uneven, highly pressured in some areas and not supported enough in others, it will bulge out of the connective tissue container like an inner tube through a worn tyre. The most visible result of this may simply be a distended abdomen, but there could also be haemorrhoids, prolapse or a hiatus hernia, as well as compression of the inter-vertebral discs.

When we examine the mechanical forces that act on the body – the pull of muscles on joints, the expanse of connective tissue and the way it organises the bones of the body – we can fall into the trap of thinking of the body as a machine. We can think of adjusting the mechanics a little in order to make it run more smoothly.

Body mechanics are very important, as anyone suffering with musculo-skeletal problems will testify, and yoga lends itself to the analysis of movement and the stresses and strains that are put on the components of movement. However, yoga also has a long history of addressing the visceral and respiratory health of the body, and these are as important as body mechanics.

The musculo-skeletal system and the respiratory system form their shapes and patterns in response to the promptings of the nervous system; how we breathe and how we move during the course of our lives will shape us, literally. And if this shape needs changing because it has lost balance and equilibrium, then the nervous system will have to change its prompting to restore equilibrium.

In yoga it is possible to address all these components within the human structure – the fluid body, the connective body and the neurological body. Through the postures of yoga we seek to bring a balance to the muscles,

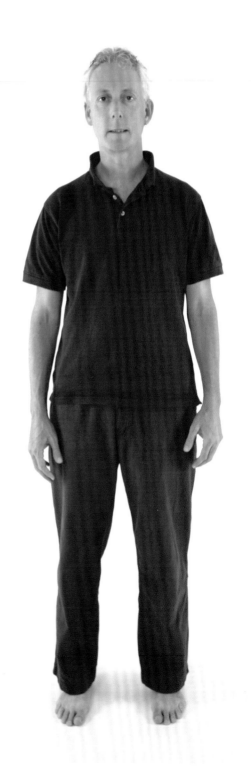

tendons and other connective tissues. Through breathing techniques we contain the fluid mass of the abdomen and pelvis, harmonising the muscles of the abdominal wall, diaphragm and pelvic floor.

Inverted poses and bandhas help to counteract the downward pressure of the gravitational force we are unable to escape. Through close attention to our body and breath we increase our awareness of, and are perhaps able to confront, the habits ingrained in our neural system.

It is not my intention to provide a comprehensive textbook of either anatomy or yoga. Rather, this is an exercise in the weaving together of the two, to create an anatomy of experience. As this book unfolds we will undoubtedly uncover some important anatomical and physiological facts, but this will be with the sole intention of building a bigger and more holistic picture. We do not experience ourselves as separate organs and discrete systems. Nor do we thrive as isolated human beings.

We experience our bodies as an integrated whole – when we experience them at all. For so much of our lives our bodies are nothing more than the vehicle that carries around our brains. Yoga enables us to redress the balance, to experience our bodies in the moment, to wake up to the details of that experience and to become interested in the way they feel and respond. We may even find that as we learn to inhabit our bodies more fully we become more fully conscious of ourselves and of our humanity, and in doing so find health.

Taking with us the most fundamental precept of all, that there is, in anatomical terms at least, no beginning, no middle and no end, we will begin where life itself began – with the sea.

We will look more closely at how we carry it around with us. To recap, we are water-based organisms. We take water in and we excrete water out. If we are punctured we leak, and if we loose too much fluid we die.

It is easy to forget that 70% of our body weight is water. The average human body has 46 litres of water constantly circulating within its connective tissue. This gravity-defying feat starts at conception and carries on until death, at which point circulation finally ceases. The very fact that fluid is pumped, sucked and percolated throughout the body without a break for our entire lives is testimony to the essential role it plays in our existence.

Circulation carries the stuff of life – oxygen and nutrition. It carries information in the form of hormones, neuro-peptides and other informational molecules, and transmits warmth from the core to the extremities. Every function of the body is dependent on the watery system of circulation for its completion. If we recognise the huge importance that fluid circulation has on our health, it must follow that anything impairing this circulation is liable to have a detrimental effect on our well-being.

As I have already pointed out, when considering circulation our first thought goes to the cardiovascular system, for this is what most people have been taught. Yet only three to three-and-a-half litres of fluid – out of 46 – is contained within the cardiovascular system. The remaining 40-odd litres are not pumped around the body by the heart. Most of the remaining fluid exists within the cells and in the tissue surrounding the cells. Some also exists as digestive juices, cerebrospinal fluid, ocular fluid, urine and so on. Like connective tissue, water permeates all parts of the human organism, but unlike connective tissue it is constantly changing its position.

If you could follow a single water molecule on its journey around the body it would start in the mouth as water drunk, and would then pass through the digestive system to be absorbed into the blood stream when it reached the colon. At some point on its journey it would leave the blood stream to enter a cell where it would be called intra-cellular fluid. It may then leave the cell and become interstitial fluid before being swept into the lymphatic vessels where it would become known as lymph.

The point is that the various systems of the body are not discrete. Water moves indiscriminately from one situation to another all the time. To understand how this can happen we must recognise the body as a series of pumps, pipes and pouches that channel, contain and squeeze their watery fluids from place to place.

Pulsation – the life force

Nature abhors stillness; everywhere there is movement and vibration. On a cosmic scale solar systems and galaxies swirl around the universe, while on our dynamic planet continents shift on their molten foundations. Even the apparent immobility of a block of steel is an illusion, for we know the atoms that provide its structure are vibrant with energetic movement.

In a living organism movement takes on another quality. Somewhere at the core of each living creature, movement becomes life and life becomes movement. The cell, the basic unit of life, is a watery structure – liquid surrounded by a delicate membrane. Fluid circulates within it, leaks into and out of it, into other cells, and out of other cells. Within this fluid are the substances needed for life; some are dissolved and some are swept along. The most important of these are oxygen, glucose and certain other nutrients, products such as carbon dioxide, hormones

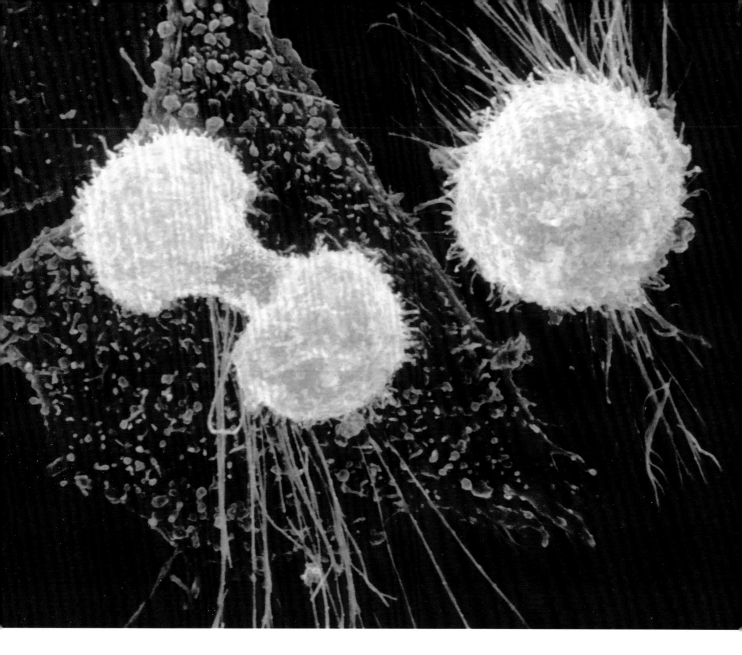

and other chemical messengers. All move with the fluid tides of the body. Within cells, tiny molecular forms called organelles process these tidal components and expel them again in a form useful to the body.

We know that some fluids follow concentrations of particles held in solution, always trying to establish a balance. If more glucose appears on one side of a cell membrane than the other, fluid will move across the membrane in an effort to dilute the more saturated side. This balancing of concentrations is complicated by the fact that cell membranes are selective in the molecules they allow through, so imbalances of particle concentrations always develop.

Water, with its own peculiar drive, always seeks to rebalance. This is the process of osmosis. But osmosis is not enough to explain the streams and currents that take place within

a cell or outside of it; some other force powers these. Each cell oscillates, vibrates in response to some inherent vitality or something given by its environment. What causes this is difficult to say, but a dead cell does not vibrate. The life of the cell is expressed through its vibration. Vibration, or pulsation, is the expression of life.

The very first human cell, formed by the meeting of sperm and ovum, is called the zygote. Pulsation and motility is in evidence from the very beginning; as the zygote divides, its division is marked by elongation and shortening, until it stretches itself in two. There is no stasis here. These divisions divide again and again and so on, until there are many thousands of cells, which together form a fluid-filled ball. This cellular sphere, the blastocyst, itself oscillates with the vitality of its cells. After a few days it embeds itself in the wall of the uterus. Layers form within the ball and something distinctive

The fluid body – an anatomy of experience

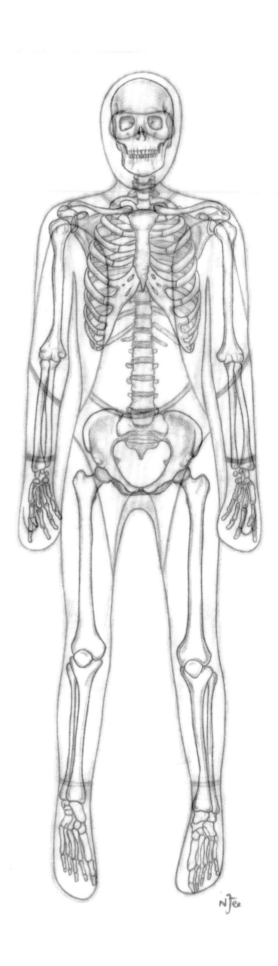

occurs; for the first time there is a difference in the type of cells that develop.

Three specific layers are formed within the blastocyst. The middle layer is known as the mesoderm, from which all the connective tissue of the body will emerge, together with the muscles, tissues, bones and fascia. The outer layer is the ectoderm, from which the nervous tissue and skin will emerge.

Many of the body's organs, including the lungs, liver, pancreas and other organs of digestion derive from the inner layer, the endoderm. Eventually the first discernible feature becomes apparent; the central layer becomes denser, and is called the notochord. This develops into the spine. After a few days a swelling appears at one end of the notochord which will become the head. At the same time other cells are developing.

Close to the head, a group of cells starts oscillating in unison, imposing a steady rhythm on the developing embryo. These pulsing cells will become the heart. The early embryonic structure is soft and fluid but gradually consolidations appear within the cellular matrix. The notochord condenses into cartilage and within these cartilaginous templates areas of ossification start to appear.

By the fifth week little growth buds develop near the top and bottom of the developing spine. These grow out of the centre forming the arms and legs, at first soft and pliable but slowly consolidating into delicate areas of bone. Humeruses and femurs appear followed by radiuses, tibias, tiny carpal and tarsal bones. Individual skull bones form within its membranous template. All this takes place in a liquid environment; there is no air to breathe, no gravity to respond to, just a soft growing form in a safe, watery embrace.

Muscles have formed, but because of the lack of gravity, movements are more akin to those of a water creature: swimming movements, expanding and contracting. Breathing is practiced as amniotic fluid is drawn into the lungs and expelled out again. At this stage of life the navel is effectively the mouth of the foetus, its source of nutrition and life.

Knowing this we can better imagine a different take on human anatomy: that of a soft, water-filled creature, a more fluid and less rigid structure; one that responds differently to gravity, and requires the sustenance of pulsation.

If we build ourselves from this viewpoint, a quite different perspective on anatomy emerges. Imagine a body filled simply with fluid; a diving suit perhaps, filled with water. The form of this body is determined by the suit, and its substance by the water. The suit itself is akin to the connective tissue of the body, the container for our watery selves.

If for a moment we forget the function of the internal organs and consider only their structural properties, we can imagine them as water-filled balloons creating form and support. We would then have a water-filled suit packed with water-filled balloons at its centre, in the large chamber of the abdomen and pelvis. Imagine too that we substitute the muscles for a kind of fine sponge drenched in and surrounded by water. Then imagine easing the bones of the body into place, inserting the foot bones into the bottom of the suit, manoeuvring the tibias and femurs into place through the muscular sponge, and placing the pelvis on top. The spine, the ribs, the arms, the shoulders and head would all then follow.

The picture we have now is not the traditional one of the bony skeleton supporting the weight of the body. Rather, the bones are embedded

The fluid body – an anatomy of experience

The evolution of breathing casts some light on the role of respiratory muscles in the modern human being

in a matrix of fluid and tissue. Bones do indeed transmit forces through the body, but the load on the bones and the joints can be reduced greatly if the surrounding fluid matrix supports them well.

Let us consider our diving suit man again and build in more carefully the thoracic and abdominal pelvic cavity. With the abdomen squeezed in, fluid would be forced both upward and downward, rather like a toothpaste tube squeezed in the middle. The suit would elongate from top to bottom, taking the attached bones with it, including the spine. Space would be created from the centre outwards, taking the load off the joints.

This actually happens every time we breathe. When we exhale we gather in around the waist and an elongation impulse, upwards and downwards, extends us and grounds us at the same time. In fact, every compartment in the body is capable of developing pressure and resisting gravity. Standing is not merely a muscular activity.

It is the interaction between the waves of pulsation pushing up and down, the bodily compartments and the diaphragms between them, that results in the internal pressure that resists gravity. Two waves interact – one to push down, one to push up. From this point of view, the organisation of fluids within the upright body is one of the vital anti-gravity mechanisms at our disposal.

In the human body fluids are contained by expanses of muscle and connective tissue. If this container is allowed to function unhindered, our bodily fluids can resist the pull of gravity. When muscular tension interferes with balanced standing, not only are these pulsations inhibited and our anti-gravity mechanism compromised, but the joints of the body are brought under

strain, with the concomitant sequela of discomfort and pain.

When we look at the body it quickly becomes clear that the major area of fluid containment is the abdominal and pelvic cavity. This area, below the diaphragm and above the pelvic floor, is one large fluid container – with the fluid held in the organs. When this area is well contained, the body receives a great deal of hydrostatic support, but when it is not contained well, collapse or strain may occur throughout the body.

At the roof of the abdominal cavity is the diaphragm, while at the floor of the pelvic cavity are the pelvic floor muscles. The deepest abdominal muscles, the transverse abdominals, comprise a vertical wall. All are voluntary muscles that are capable, like any other skeletal muscles, of developing habits. However, the primary function provided by these muscles is breathing.

The breath, therefore, has a significant role in fluid support and in our response to gravity. To understand how, we need to understand the mechanics of breathing. The evolution of breathing casts some light on the role of respiratory muscles in the modern human being.

The evolution of breathing

Lizards have a problem; to move forwards they need to employ sideways movements of the spine similar to that used by a fish swimming through water. For this movement a lizard must use the muscles that control its ribs. This is very inconvenient for the lizard which needs these muscles in order to breathe.

A lizard cannot run and breathe at the same time without getting puffed out very quickly. Lizards tend not to breathe when they run, but stand still afterwards and breathe by expansion and contraction of their rib cage. Breathing

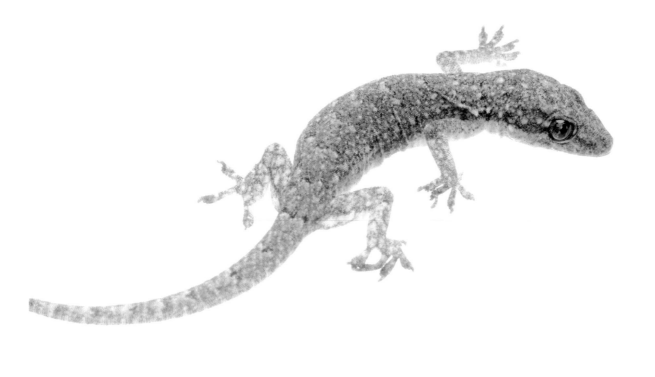

like this, with just the ribs, is comparatively inefficient; when pressure falls in the rib cage, not only is air sucked into the lungs, but the organs are sucked up as well, occupying space that could otherwise be occupied by an inflated lung.

Some dinosaurs, primarily the upright, two-legged therapods started to overcome this problem with the development of a primitive diaphragm. Crocodiles developed a similar rudimentary diaphragm. This helped hold the organs in place as well as enabling these creatures to run and breathe at the same time.

Modern mammals have taken this development further: the diaphragm is more muscular and pushes the organs down as it contracts. In mammals, the lizard's lumbar ribs have been replaced by strong abdominal muscles which enable fully functioning diaphragmatic respiration while running, allowing the ribs to be used partly for their locomotor role. In four-legged animals the lumbar spine can now flex and extend to improve the speed of running. Think of the running cheetah or galloping horse,

and the flexion and extension that comes from their abdominal / lumbar regions.

The development of the diaphragm and the necessity of a reciprocal abdomen solved one problem but created another; an abdomen large enough to respond to a strong muscular diaphragm meant, as already mentioned, the loss of the reptilian lumbar ribs and the support they provided to the abdominal area. This support has to be provided instead by the abdominal muscles, muscles that also have to breathe. We can start to see now how intimately linked support and breathing are.

By becoming bipedal, humans have freed themselves a stage further; with the arms no longer needed for locomotion, the ribs can assume a larger respiratory role than they have in quadrupeds. However, when we support ourselves on our arms we can often find the ribs reverting to their postural role and becoming fixed. This complex interplay between movement, support and the breath needs close study if we are to shed light on its optimum function.

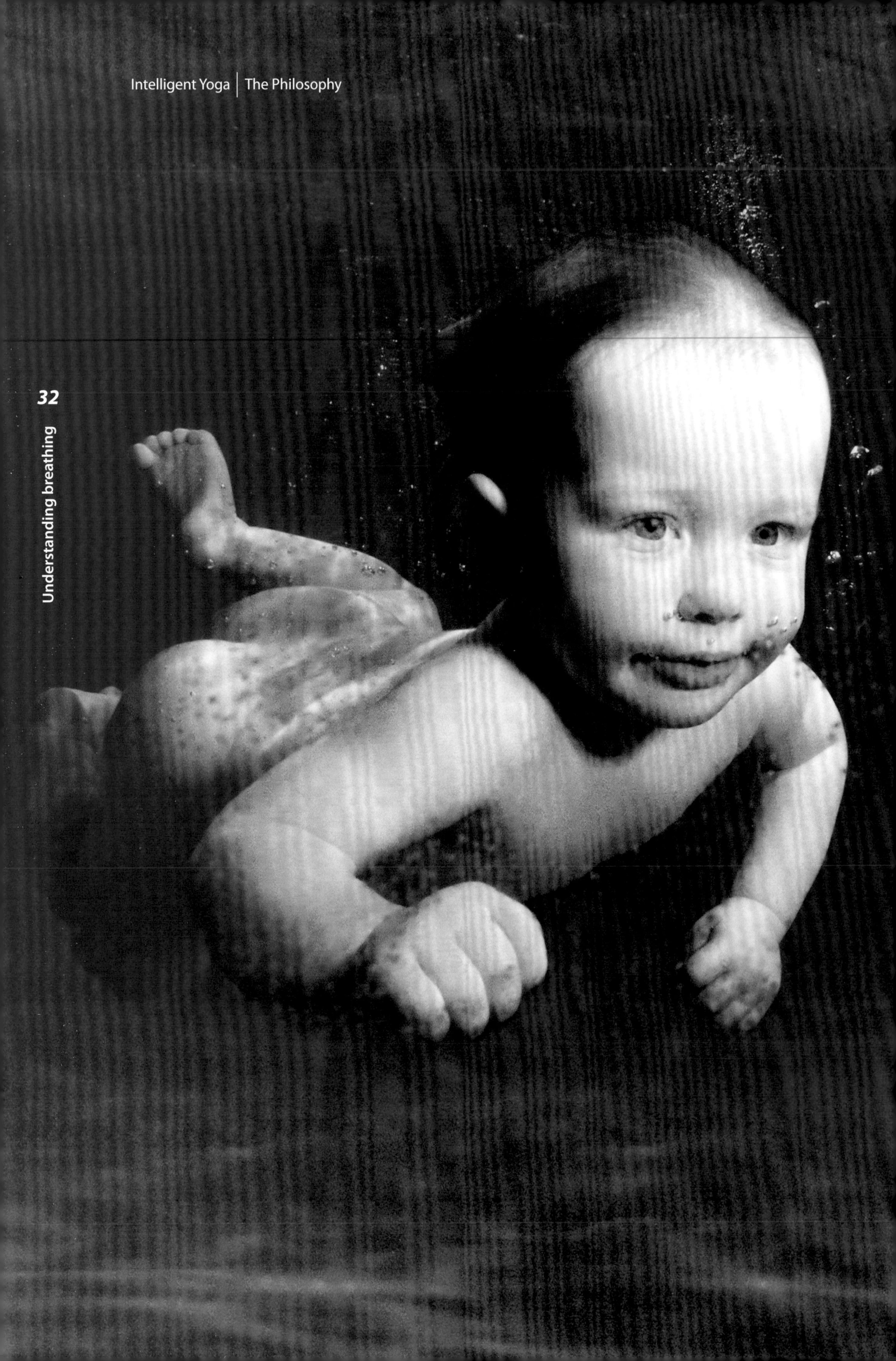

CHAPTER THREE
Understanding breathing

To develop an understanding of this vital function of the body, we need to recognise the scope of its effects. Responses to the breath are not limited to the rib cage. Indeed our breath engages both the thoracic and abdominal cavities as well as the muscles that form their base, namely the diaphragm and the pelvic floor. These areas at the core of the body are related not just in structure, through their proximity, but also in function. In fact they are so closely related functionally that it is impossible to make sense of one without reference to the others.

The human body, as we have seen, is made up of pouches, chambers and tubes, most of which are fluid-filled and all of which are surrounded by muscular layers and connective tissue. How these tissues and muscles contain the fluid-filled structures of the body goes a long way to shaping a person's posture – their upright response to gravity. Tubes or pouches confined by muscles create pressure; muscles that constrict and then release sequentially, create circulation.

In his 1985 book *Emotional Anatomy*[2], Stanley Keleman captures this aspect of our nature perfectly: "Standing is not a mechanical event – bones resting on bones supporting weight on the earth. Nor is it achieved through the tonus of anti-gravitational muscles. Standing is a vertical pulsatory pattern, a pumping action. It is a rhythmical pattern of expansion and contraction that moves excitatory fluids through space. In standing we learn to sustain the pressures that make for an effective human pump."

When we examine the thorax and the abdomino-pelvic cavity, we are looking at the two biggest chambers in the body. The upper chamber, the thorax, is directly related to breathing; pressure changes within the thorax allow respiration to take place. Being air filled, it can be considered a pneumatic structure.

The lower chamber, comprising the abdomen and pelvis, is responsible for expulsion; pressure changes here enable excretion, urination and birth. The lower chamber is fluid filled and can therefore be considered a hydraulic structure.

The two chambers are separated by the diaphragm, a tendino-muscular sheet that provides a floor to the thorax and a ceiling to the abdomen. Each chamber is capable of changing its size by constricting or relaxing the muscles surrounding it. However, the change in pressure in one chamber will always affect the pressure in the other via the diaphragm. This would be a relatively straightforward mechanical process if the diaphragm were a passive membrane, but clearly it is not. The diaphragm is a muscle capable of changing its shape and size, and is therefore able to influence the pressure in both chambers simultaneously.

The thorax – the upper chamber

Mechanically nature was faced with a problem. Air will only move from an area of high pressure to an area of low pressure; it will only move into the lungs if the pressure inside them is lower than the pressure on the outside.

It is relatively easy to increase pressure in a chamber; you simply tighten muscles around its circumference and the pressure inside goes up. But in order to draw air into the lungs the inside pressure needs to fall. The chamber has to expand.

Given that the only tools we have to change our size and shape naturally are muscles, and given that these can only shorten and contract, nature faced a significant challenge to its ingenuity. Its solution was the rib cage; thanks to our elaborately shaped ribs and the way they hinge at the thoracic vertebrae, humans – indeed all mammals – are able to expand their thorax. In so doing, the internal pressure is lowered and, via the basic physical law of pressure gradients, air is then pushed into the lungs.

While this seems straightforward, it is worth noting that lung tissue is surrounded by a double serous membrane which secretes a slippery fluid. The inner membrane, the visceral pleura, attaches to the lung tissue while the outer membrane, the parietal pleura, attaches to the inside of the rib cage.

The serous fluid allows friction-free movement between the two membranes, which should remain in contact. When the thoracic cavity expands at the widening and lifting of the ribs, the parietal pleura has to go with it. This creates a potential vacuum between the membranes, which demands that the visceral pleura fills the space and moves with it.

Elevating the rib cage

The rib elevator muscles are varied, with some at the front, some at the back and some at the sides. The upper ribs are elevated by a group of muscles called the scalenes. These small neck muscles have their origin at the cervical vertebrae and insert into the first and second ribs. Now considered primary respiratory muscles, their involvement in breathing – if over-used – can transmit tension to the neck.

The serratus posterior superior, which originate on the spinous processes of C7 to T3 vertebrae, helps elevate the second to fifth ribs. The small levatores costarum, originating on the transverse processes of the first eleven thoracic vertebrae, and inserting into the tubercle of the rib below, also helps elevate the rib it is attached to. It is probable that the external intercostals do play some part in elevating the ribs, but current thinking suggests that their role is more postural – helping to maintain an appropriate space between each rib during respiration and movement.

Because of the differences in the way the ribs attach to the spine, the lower ribs are lifted out sideways, in what is sometimes referred to as a bucket handle action. The upper ribs and the breast bone elevate differently, moving forwards and upwards, in a pump handle action. As we breathe in the lower rib cage tends to widen, while the upper rib cage deepens.

Passive exhalation is often believed to occur simply because of the recoil of the elastic elements of inhalation – mainly the connective tissue of the lungs with the lower ribs fixed largely by the quadratus lumborum below. Recently, however, electromyographic evidence suggests that exhalation is never completely passive, as the diaphragm maintains a tone to slow down the rate of elastic recoil in the

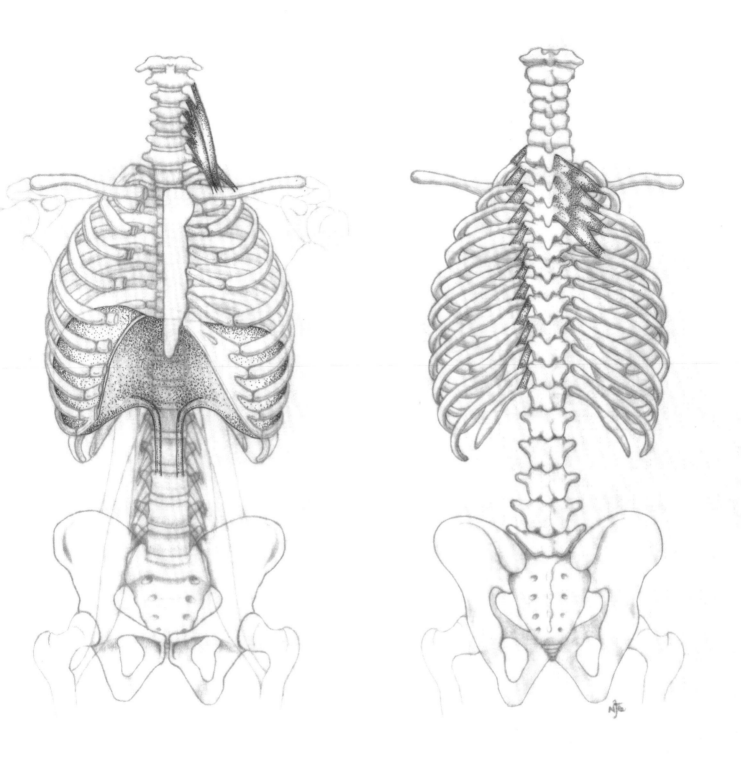

respiratory tissues. Without this diaphragmatic control, the lungs would spring back too quickly, forcing air out in an uncontrolled way.

The diaphragm

This musculo-tendonous dome forms the floor of the thorax and separates the thoracic cavity from the abdomen. Openings in the diaphragm allow the passage of the major blood vessels, lymphatics, nerves and the oesophagus. At the apex of the dome is the central tendon from which bands of muscle fibres radiate out to the periphery, attaching to the deep surfaces of the costal cartilages and the tips of the 11th

and 12th ribs. At the back, the dome extends further with fibres reaching down to attach at the front of the first, second and third lumbar vertebrae. There is a fascial continuum between the diaphragm and the psoas and quadratus lumborum, by means of the left and right crura. When the diaphragm contracts, the central tendon is pulled down, much like a piston sliding in a pump, and this increases the vertical diameter of the thorax.

The descent of the diaphragm however is opposed; the mediastinum, the oesophagus, aorta and vena cava, which all pass through the diaphragm, stretch only to the extent of their

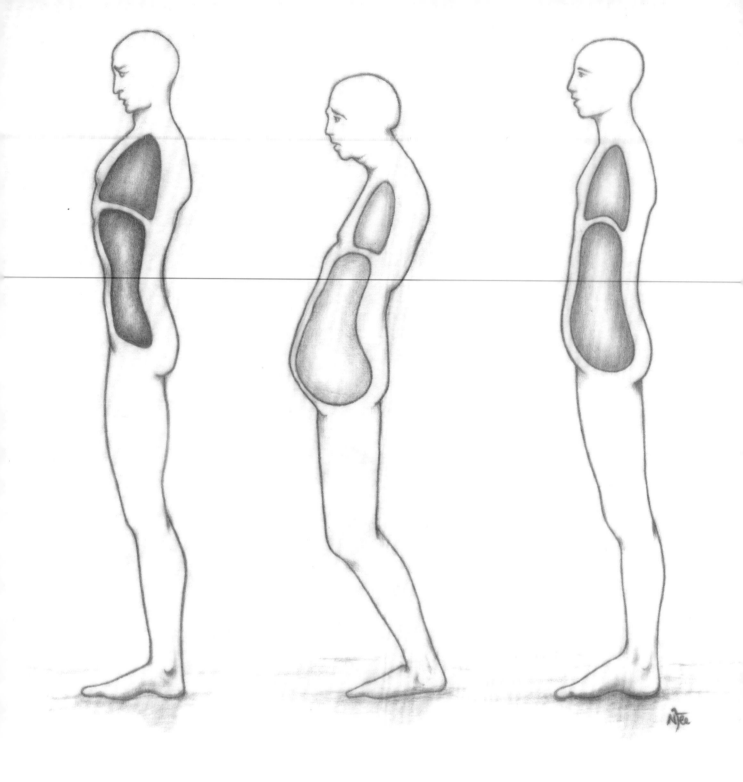

elastic limits. Resistance is provided too by the abdominal organs from below.

When the diaphragm can descend no further, the central tendon becomes fixed and the muscle fibres, now acting from the edge of the central tendon, act instead to elevate the lower ribs. Via this mechanism, the descent of the diaphragm not only increases the vertical dimension of the thorax but also widens it, increasing its capacity both vertically and laterally. In fact, the diaphragm is quite capable of elevating the entire rib cage; if the lower ribs are pulled up by it will, by virtue of their attachment to the costal cartilage, lift that as well.

The lower chamber: the abdominal and pelvic cavity

We have observed that air is drawn into the lungs by the increased size of the thoracic cavity, achieved by the expansion of the rib cage and the descent of the diaphragm. We have also discovered that as the diaphragm descends it moves against the incompressible fluid content of the abdomen and pelvis. This in turn puts pressure on the walls of this cavity, the anterior abdominal wall and the pelvic floor (the lumbar spine too, of course).

During exhalation the diaphragm rises, drawing the abdominal contents with it. The pelvic floor and abdominal wall follow, inwards and upwards. This synergic movement between the diaphragm, abdomen and pelvic floor is very significant in terms of the core fluid support of the body. To understand this relationship we must take a look at the structure and function of this lower chamber as well as its response to the breath.

The abdomen

In many ways the abdomen is a relatively simple structure, as its main function is one of stricture. The deep abdominal muscle that forms the wall of the abdomen and pelvis, the transverse abdominus, is ideally suited for this task.

The transverse abdominus forms an almost continuous structure with the diaphragm above and blends with the muscles of the inner wall of the pelvis below. With its horizontally aligned fibres, contraction of this muscle raises pressure in the abdomen and pelvis. This increase in intra-abdominal pressure is needed firstly as a means for expulsion – for excretion, vomiting, coughing and giving birth.

Secondly, it provides support. This becomes quite obvious when we instinctively brace the abdomen when trying to lift a heavy object, and in so doing form an hydraulic column in order to protect the spine. In everyday life, support is also provided by the relative tensions of the abdominal muscular wall. However, some clarification is needed about the relative roles played by the muscles of this wall. They can be divided into two main groups, those used for moving the skeleton, and those used to support the abdominal contents. The muscles used to move the skeleton are the external and internal obliques, and the rectus abdominus. The transverse abdominus supports the abdominal contents as well as increasing intra-abdominal pressure, as previously described.

The pelvic floor

More complex in structure is the pelvic floor. In women particularly the pelvic floor has to accommodate two paradoxical actions. Firstly it provides the floor to the abdomen and pelvis, so it needs the strength to be able to resist the pressure exerted from above. It also provides the passage for birth and must therefore be "giving" enough to accommodate a baby. These dual roles would probably be completely incompatible were it not for the release of certain hormones during pregnancy and birth which render the supporting tissues more malleable.

In terms of its structure, the pelvic floor centres around the perineal body, a fibro muscular node between the anus and vagina, which provides attachment to eight muscles. In terms of support, the transverse perinei, which are both deep and superficial, run from the perineal body to the inner surface of the two ischeal tuberosities or sitting bones. The sphincter ani surrounds the anus, while the bulbospongiosus surrounds the vagina, making a saggital connection between the coccyx and pubic bone. Together these muscles form a cruciform structure at the base of the pelvic floor.

Below this, and also connected to the perineal body, are the levator ani, two large, flat muscles attached to the inner surface of the pubic bone and to the ischium. At the back of the pelvic floor, at the same depth as the levator ani, the coccygeus runs from the sacrum and coccyx and inserts into the ischeal spine.

This is a very tough muscle, blending with the sacrotuberous ligament. On the inner surface of these two muscles, adding strength to the pelvic floor, is a layer of fascia sometimes described as "the wallpaper of the pelvis". Although there are other small muscles, and another deeper layer of fascia, these muscles form the principle

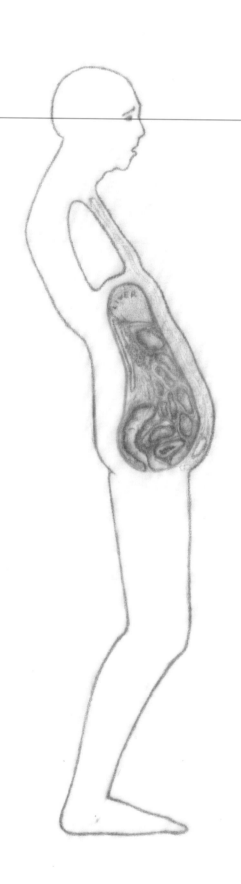

supporting structures. Both the levator ani and the coccygeus have the effect of lifting the pelvic floor when contracted, resulting in the closing of the anus, urethra and the vagina in women. It seems that these two muscles maintain a "postural tone" most of the time.

Imbalance in the chambers

Although the pelvic floor is the base of the pelvis and therefore receives much of the weight of the abdominal contents, there are two mitigating factors. The first is the shape of the lower pelvic organs, particularly the uterus and the bladder. As these are spherical, much of their weight is distributed to the surrounding muscles and ligaments. The second is thoracic suction which, as Jean Pierre Barral explains in *Visceral Manipulation*[3], occurs with the upward release of the diaphragm during exhalation: "The supra-diaphragmatic pressure is lower than the sub-diaphragmatic pressure, so that the contents of the abdominal cavity are in effect suspended from the diaphragm. The force of gravity in the abdominal cavity acts against this upward force. The organs closest to the diaphragm are most sensitive to this effect, and the further we descend into the abdomen, the more it is attenuated. The weight of the liver for example which is approximately 2kg, is effectively diminished by more than half thanks to the attraction effect created by pressure differentials."

It is of course possible to expand the thorax without using the ribs, as we do when we breathe abdominally. Here the diaphragm descends much further pushing down on the abdominal contents and negating much of the suspensory effect. Ideally, with a healthy balance between the rib cage, the diaphragm and the abdomino-pelvic cavity, the upper chamber is expansive enough to enable this general drawing up of the abdominal contents. However imbalance can develop, particularly if tension in the diaphragm accumulates. Shortening in the diaphragm will cause it to tighten downwards against the abdominal contents, increasing pressure on the abdominal wall and pelvic floor. The notion of chronic tension in the diaphragm is difficult to prove, but patterns of respiration change when we are anxious and the excursion of the diaphragm tends to diminish. Like other skeletal muscles, shortening happens when a range of movement is regularly curtailed.

This reciprocally weakens these muscles, which lose their ability to resist pressure from above. The result for the individual is not only the ubiquitous pear shape that develops in later middle years, but also more insidious problems. Vertical support is lost, so the lumbar spine may come under strain. Thoracic suction is also lost, so organs can migrate downwards. When the shape of the cavity changes, the position of the organs also has to change. The kidneys, the stomach and the entire small intestine are supported principally by the pressure of the container they are in. Many other organs hang directly from the diaphragm. If the diaphragm moves down, they go with it. The shape and size of all hollow organs in the pelvis and abdomen are determined in response to the external pressure exerted on it. If intra-abdominal pressure is increased chronically, the hollow organs will tend to compress. If intra-abdominal pressure falls, they will expand.

Clearly the relative position of the diaphragm and abdominal wall will affect the placement of the more mobile organs. One can speculate that an organ, lets us say the transverse colon, will function better when appropriately positioned than when it is sagging. It seems reasonable to assume that the better placed an organ is, the better it will function. Downward pressure

from the diaphragm will push on the pelvic floor which may contribute to problems such as stress incontinence and prolapse.

In order to address these symptoms or, perhaps more realistically, to prevent them before they develop, we cannot merely look at the structure that is in trouble and try to repair it. If our concern is with the integrity of the pelvic floor, it is of little use just doing pelvic floor exercises. The pelvic floor has come under stress because of a breakdown in the balance of the two chambers, so to improve the situation this balance must be restored.

One individual who took a great interest in this aspect of human health was an orthopaedic surgeon working at the first half of the twentieth century. In his book *Body Mechanics and Health*[4] Joel E. Goldthwaite outlines his belief that many chronic diseases are caused by the "mal position of the organs and viscera". He backs up his belief with many fascinating case histories, and with X-ray evidence of organ positions before and after treatment.

One of Goldthwaite's principal aims was to release chronically tightened diaphragms, for he believed this was central in restoring better health and vitality. His methods were crude by our reckoning – using plaster casts and leather corsets to hold his patients into the position he felt was beneficial – but he achieved extraordinary results. His book illustrates how a tightly packed body can become disorganised when its shape changes.

It is dangerous to read too much into the work of one man working in the early part of the last century. However, before the discovery of the "miracle drugs" of the latter part of the 20th century there was a large movement of health professionals who took an interest in how exercise, posture and breathing could improve health.

The innocent breath

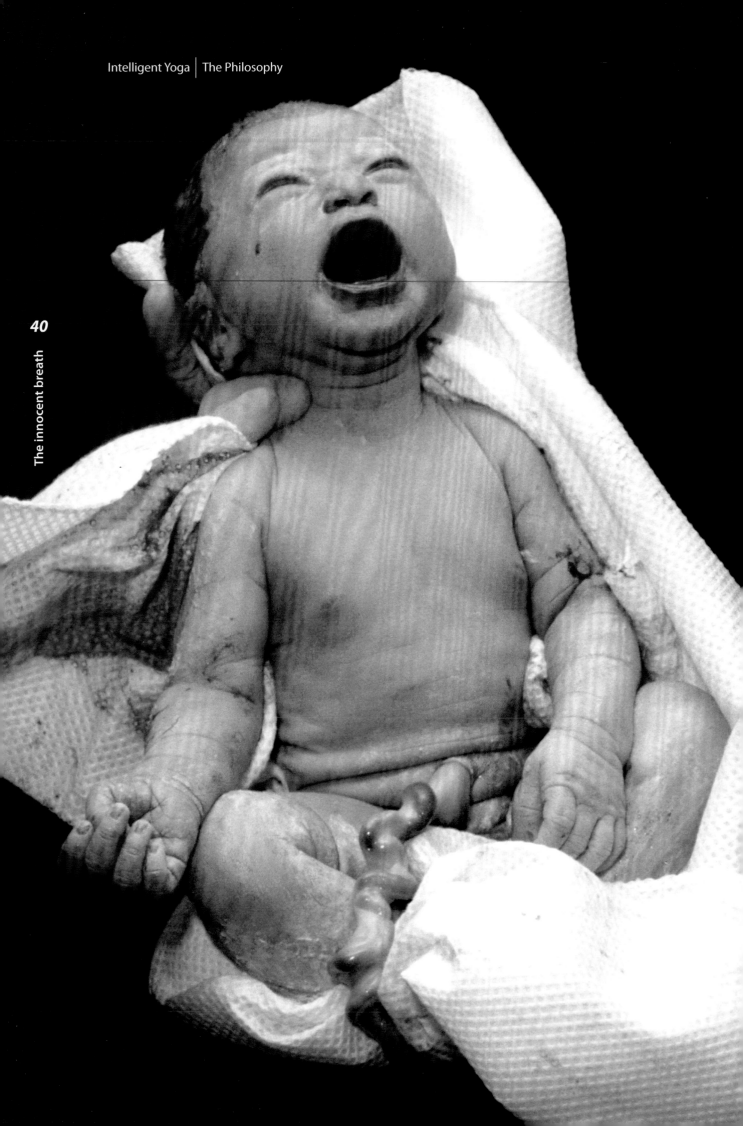

CHAPTER FOUR
The innocent breath

Breathing happens, we don't have to think about it. Between 10 and 14 times a minute we breathe in and breathe out. Breathing is a natural function, regulated from centres in the medulla and pons of the lower brain. In the baby and young child the interplay between the thoracic and abdominal chambers is obvious and innocent. Almost all parts of the body respond naturally to the breath. As we get older, however, the dynamics can change.

All the muscles of respiration and those of the abdominal and pelvic cavity are voluntary, and like all voluntary muscles they can be habituated. The respiratory muscles seem particularly prone to habituation. This is not entirely surprising given that breathing is one of the first things that changes in response to emotional fluctuations. Any sustained emotional pattern will be reflected in a sustained change in breathing. Changes in respiration eventually change the shape of the thorax, and changes in the shape of the thorax eventually change the shape of the lower chamber. With this change the function of the lower chamber may be compromised.

To understand why such changes occur we must recognise the different influences that act on the breath. In normal, quiet respiration our breathing is regulated by a default setting in the respiratory centres of the lower brain.

When we are asleep the respiratory centres send impulses down the phrenic and intercostal nerves, causing the diaphragm and rib elevator muscles respectively, to contract approximately once every five seconds.

It is important from a survival point of view that this rhythm can be overridden. If we fall into water we must be able to hold our breath for a certain period of time. Talking and singing require modification to the normal respiratory pattern achieved through cortical control – the higher centres of the brain inhibiting the commands from the lower centres.

Another influence arises from the chemical receptors in the arterial system and the ventricles of the brain. These chemical receptors are very sensitive to levels of carbon dioxide in the blood and cerebro-spinal fluid. If carbon dioxide levels rise, the receptors recognise this and inform the respiratory centres to increase the breathing rate. This allows the excess build-up of carbon dioxide to be blown off until blood levels are back to normal. Left to their own devices and a constant environment these regulatory systems would keep our breathing trouble free.

Our evolved cortex

Our environment is not constant, it is ever changing. Part of the success of the human species is its ability to survive in a changing environment. We are able to adapt because of

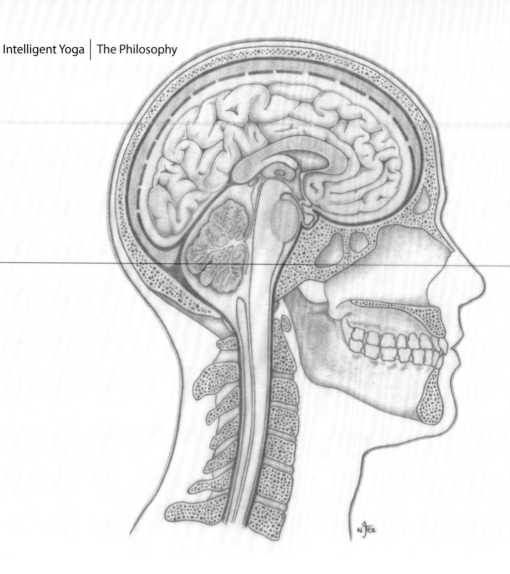

ABOVE
The complex
nature of our
cerebral cortex
has evolved
beyond that
of any other
animal

the remarkably complex nature of the cerebral cortex, the part of the brain that has evolved beyond the level of that of any other animal on the planet. With it we are able to inhibit our lower brain centres more fully than any other species. Consequently we do not act like animals any more. We have gained the advantages of a co-operative, sophisticated society. The down side is that our sub-cortical functions can be interfered with; the breath, which has a direct link to the cortex, is especially vulnerable to this.

Consider the "startle reflex", a reflex most animals have when confronted with unexpected danger. This enables them to freeze their position, and to still or quieten their breathing so that maximum attention can be focused on any possible threat. In the natural world the threat passes and breathing and muscular activity return to normal. In the complexity of our modern world this too often is not the case for humans, as perceived threats can exist for weeks, months, or even years.

Over a period of time, these constant cortical

interferences become a new default setting; a new pattern is established that has chronic health implications. Such new patterns can come from many sources, not only from the startle reflex. Social conditioning for example may instil in us a way of holding the body that alters the breathing pattern, perhaps encouraging us to stand with our chest puffed out, military style, or with our tummy held in.

We may have a job that constantly folds us in a particular way, restricting breathing in a certain area of the body. No other free animal on the planet has such influences acting upon it, nor the ability – courtesy of the cortex – to "accommodate" these influences.

Redressing the balance

Yoga, if practised with this intention provides an opportunity to optimise the way the upper and lower chambers of the trunk work. We have established that what happens in one chamber directly impacts on the other. We know the primary function of the upper chamber is respiration, so it makes sense that the rib cage and diaphragm are free and responsive enough for breathing to remain un-compromised.

It is equally important that activity in the lower chamber does not interfere with the efficiency of the thorax; this lower chamber needs to provide both postural and visceral support. It needs to be able to increase pressure enough for expulsive efforts, but must not interfere unnecessarily with the breath.

There are techniques in yoga for redressing the balance between the upper and lower chambers. Learning to release the exhalation fully helps release the diaphragm, preventing the build up of tension. The bandhas exert a strong resistance to the downward pull of the diaphragm. Mula bandha – lifting up the muscles of the pelvic floor – tones the pelvic floor and the lower abdominal muscles, while Uddiyana bandha – lifting the diaphragm while pulling the upper abdominal muscles back towards the spine through the expansion of the rib cage – causes the diaphragm to be pulled strongly upwards, sucking both the abdomen, its contents, and the pelvic floor with it. This can play a part in preventing the positional displacement and compression suffered by the abdominal and pelvic organs. If we add to this the practice of *kapalabhati* (forced exhalation with a passive inhalation) we strengthen the transverse abdominals and the pelvic floor, while the diaphragm is simultaneously encouraged to release.

Between them these three yoga techniques are ideal for helping counteract the effect of gravity and diaphragmatic tension, both of which take their toll on the upright human body as we age.

However, when we consider the implications of these muscular patterns, the virtue of abdominal breathing, often favoured in yoga teaching, comes into question.

While it is true to say that abdominal or diaphragmatic breathing is the least strenuous way to breathe, and so is well suited to relaxation, it may actually create long-term problems if it is encouraged as the preferred way of breathing all the time.

Abdominal breathing doesn't provide the necessary upright support we need in standing or sitting; some element of rib breathing is useful in the upright position. It is also true that the current trend of pulling the navel in towards the spine, or maintaining bandhas during yoga practice is also counter-productive, as this interferes with breathing. The balance between support and breathing is a delicate one, and it needs to be understood that breathing changes in response to the body's need for support. For example when lying on our backs there is no muscular support needed for the spine so the abdomen relaxes and we are belly breathers. When on all fours there is, as with all quadrupeds, a risk that the spine might sag with gravity creating compressive problems and wear at the facet joints. To prevent this happening some tension in the abdominals occurs reflexly to support the spine, which shifts breathing more into the ribs. This happens continuously as we move about our daily tasks; when the spine needs support there is a reflex tightening in the abdomen and breathing has to adapt. When the spine doesn't need support the abdomen should relax, enabling us to revert to abdominal breathing.

Above all, breathing needs to be responsive and adaptable. There is no right way to breathe. There is only breathing appropriate for the particular situation an individual finds themselves in. Breathing needs to respond to

The skeletal muscular system is the only part of the body that responds to our conscious volition

variations in posture, to our emotions, and to our oxygen demand; it can only do this if the entire respiratory system is flexible and reactive.

The neural body

Fluid circulation driven by pulsation is the life force of every living organism. Without it the organism will die. With the exception of cellular motility, which occurs throughout the body, we can see that all other expressions of pulsation – the heartbeat, the movement of the diaphragm, the circulation of the cerebral fluid – occur deep within the body. It is obvious too that they are all involuntary, continuing the tireless task of pulsation no matter what we do or think.

In human development we see the creation of the first cell, the zygote; we see its rhythmic expansions and contractions. We see that these elongations eventually lead to its division and the creation of the blastocyst, itself a swelling and shrinking mass. We see the development of the embryo, then the foetus, and we see this tiny young life form floating and swimming in its watery environment. Science allows us to observe this development at close quarters, but for the growing child it is largely an unconscious process with few, if any, concerns beyond feeding and movement.

After 40 weeks a massive change occurs: the baby is born. At this moment two hugely significant events take place. For the first time the baby is confronted with the force of gravity; no longer floating in its watery womb, it can suddenly feel the weight of its limbs. Muscles will have to strengthen in order to move these limbs against gravity.

Also, for the first time breathing becomes a matter of urgency. The mother no longer supplies oxygen via the umbilical cord; the diaphragm will now have to work unceasingly to draw oxygen

into the body. The earliest developments of the muscular and respiratory systems occur at the same time, and from this very first moment they will inevitably influence each other.

As the muscular system grows in sophistication and gradually submits to the will of the cortex, the divisions of the nervous system become more apparent. On the inside of the body we have the motility of the autonomic system, the core processes of life, while on the outside we have the developing muscular system, moving in accordance with the will of the individual. In effect we have an inner pulsation keeping the body alive, and an outer muscular container moving us around.

This inner and outer distinction is important to emphasise. The skeletal muscular system is the only part of the body that responds to our conscious volition. Everything else in the body – the organs and circulatory system – function autonomically. The one significant exception is the diaphragm, which forms a bridge between the conscious and the unconscious, responding to both voluntary and autonomic control.

The developing motor system

When a baby is born its motor control is almost nil; it is impossible for a baby to do anything it wants. Indeed, it may not even know what it wants, other than to survive. To help it do this, the nervous system is partially "hard-wired"' at birth. The breath and the heartbeat occur automatically, but this is not enough to ensure survival. The baby also needs to eat, and so it arrives with a rooting instinct, an ability to nuzzle in search of the nipple and, once it finds it, to suck. In fact, the instinct to suck is so strong that anything placed near the baby's mouth will initiate a sucking response. The voluntary muscles of the mouth come pre-programmed.

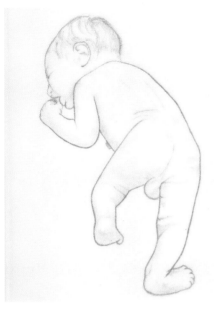

The Galant reflex: causes one-sided contraction of the trunk muscles and thus initiates the movement needed for creeping and crawling. It is similar to that used by amphibians. Eventually, these patterns of movement are used for walking.

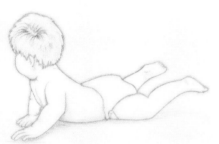

The extensor reflex: a baby develops tonic extensor reflexes which it uses initially just for its head and neck. From about three months however, the upper thoracic spine starts to extend; then by eight months most babies have developed full spinal extension.

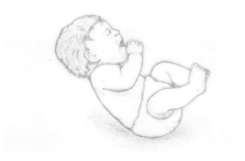

The flexor response: a newly born baby cannot lift its head, and so flexion starts at the hip; put a new born on its back and this hip flexion is immediately evident. By three months some control of head and neck flexion is apparent, and by four months this is usually integrated into an entire body flexion pattern similar to that evident in the boat postures.

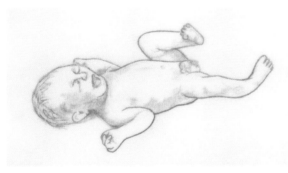

The crossed extensor reflex: makes one leg flex while the other extends. This, combined with the Galant reflex, helps with movements such as crawling and is of course vital for walking.

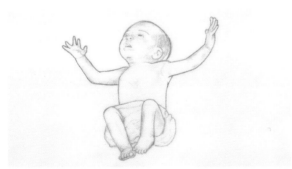

The moro reflex: is widely believed to be present prior to birth. It is a fear reflex and some experts consider it to be the precursor to the startle reflex.

We humans are locked into a constant dialogue with our surroundings. Successful living depends on our ability to interact

These are the survival reflexes without which a baby would soon die.

A reflex is any specific, predictable response that is not under the control of the conscious mind, but is elicited by a particular stimulus.

The muscular system also has more general reflexes, more survival programmes, albeit ones active in the longer term. These are reflexes that help co-ordinate the muscular system in response to gravity. They develop the sequential strength in the muscles needed for locomotion.

The importance of these motor reflexes is clear from the following quotation from *A Basis for Sensorimotor Development – Normal and Abnormal*[5], by Mary R Fiorentino: "At birth, the body is under the unopposed control of the lower centres of the central nervous system, which basically generates involuntary reflex movements and postures…. the body responds mechanically and automatically to a number of influences, such as head and body position. This affects changes in muscle tone, which then affects posture and/or movement in a number of consistent patterns termed 'primitive reflexes.'"

As the nervous system matures, these primitive reflexes contribute to the development of more complex movements, so some are worth exploring in a little more depth:

Babies express the moro reflex by drawing up their legs and spreading their arms wide. Its initiation is due to any sudden change: exteroceptive, proprioceptive, vestibular or auditory. It is generally replaced by the startle reflex by around four to six months.

One can better understand the function of the moro reflex when its context is considered. A helpless infant would need to be lifted or carried away in the presence of danger. Drawing up the legs would protect the abdomen, while reaching out with the arms facilitates being carried, a useful response for a helpless baby.

Reflexes need to be well integrated and balanced with each other in order for good motor function to develop. Interestingly many of these early reflex responses have their counterpart in yoga postures, particularly the extensor and flexor reflexes.

As we have seen, these reflexes are not cortically controlled. They are pre-programmed in the lower centres of the brain to enable the child to co-ordinate the complex movement patterns necessary for healthy motor functions.

However, at the same time the development of the cortex is continuing apace. As the reflexes we have just described begin to enable movement, the child also develops the desire to move. He or she may want to follow the movements of a parent or, later, to pick up a toy. Ideally reflexes enable the will to be acted upon.

The desire for movement integrates the reflex responses into functions such as crawling, creeping, sitting and eventually standing and walking. How successful this progression is will depend to a large extent on the emotional climate in which a child is growing. A safe, loving environment will provide the ideal background for integrated motor development. On the other hand, if the needs of the child are not met, it is likely that there will be some response to this in the body.

Anxiety and fear arise in an uncertain world. If a baby is not fed when it is hungry or is not comforted when it is unhappy, anxiety will develop.

The muscular system is the only system through which this anxiety can be expressed, and so the muscular system will inevitably exhibit change. If the anxiety is only transient the muscular system will relax again. If it continues, aberrant muscular patterns may develop.

Scientific opinion has changed recently regarding those movements designated reflexes, and towards what reflexes support. The view I have outlined here is at odds somewhat with a more modern perspective. However this is mainly with respect to terminology rather than what babies do. What I am setting out to explain is that these movements do occur in nearly all babies on a repeated basis, which implies that the spine is adapted for them. Whether they are termed locomotor flexes, primitive reflexes or postural reactions, as some authorities would have it, is in this context immaterial. For a fuller understanding of childhood motor development I recommend reading the book *Infant Motor Development*[6] by Jan P Piek.

Neurological responses to life

Obviously this is not just a problem for infants. Rather it is something that confronts us every day of our lives. Our responses to the world we live in will be reflected in the muscular patterning of our bodies. Inappropriate muscular response is invariably a reaction to stress of one form or another: we do not tighten our muscles because we are happy or relaxed.

The severity with which we tense our muscles will depend on the nature of the stress. It is quite appropriate, as a first response to a perceived threat, to be still and alert in order to assess the danger. At a job interview we may well become a little tense as we try to anticipate what is to come. When the interview is over we may sag with relief as the tension dissolves.

Living as we do in an uncertain world we are well designed for such eventualities. During time spent in an alert state we tighten our muscles and make shallow our breathing. Our digestion slows down and our heartbeat is raised. These profound physiological changes serve to increase our capacity to deal with the unexpected.

As long as this state is temporary all is fine. If the threat is continued, becoming chronic, then these patterns start to become fixed and our health may suffer as a consequence.

Problems run deeper than the muscular tension, aches and pains that we all recognise. When our outer bodies are rigid with tension, this will impact on the concomitant inner contractions. The body's natural rhythms become blocked. The depth to which we do this depends largely on the state of fear or stress encountered. We humans are locked into a constant dialogue with our surroundings. Successful living depends on our ability to interact. In his book *The Stress of Life*[7], Hans Selye makes this point well: "Life is largely a process of adaptation to circumstances in which we exist. A perennial give and take has been going on between living matter and its inanimate surroundings, between one living being and another, ever since the dawn of life in prehistoric oceans. The secret of health and happiness lies in successful adjustment to the ever-changing conditions on this globe; the penalties for failure in this great process of adaptation are disease and unhappiness."

Selye develops this view with an eye to the individual when he goes on to say: "There is another type of evolution which takes place in every person during his own lifetime, from birth to death: this adaptation to the stress of and strains of everyday existence. Through the constant interplay between his mental and bodily reactions, man has it in his power to influence this second type of evolution to a considerable extent, especially if he understands its mechanism and has enough willpower to act according to the dictates of the human intellect."

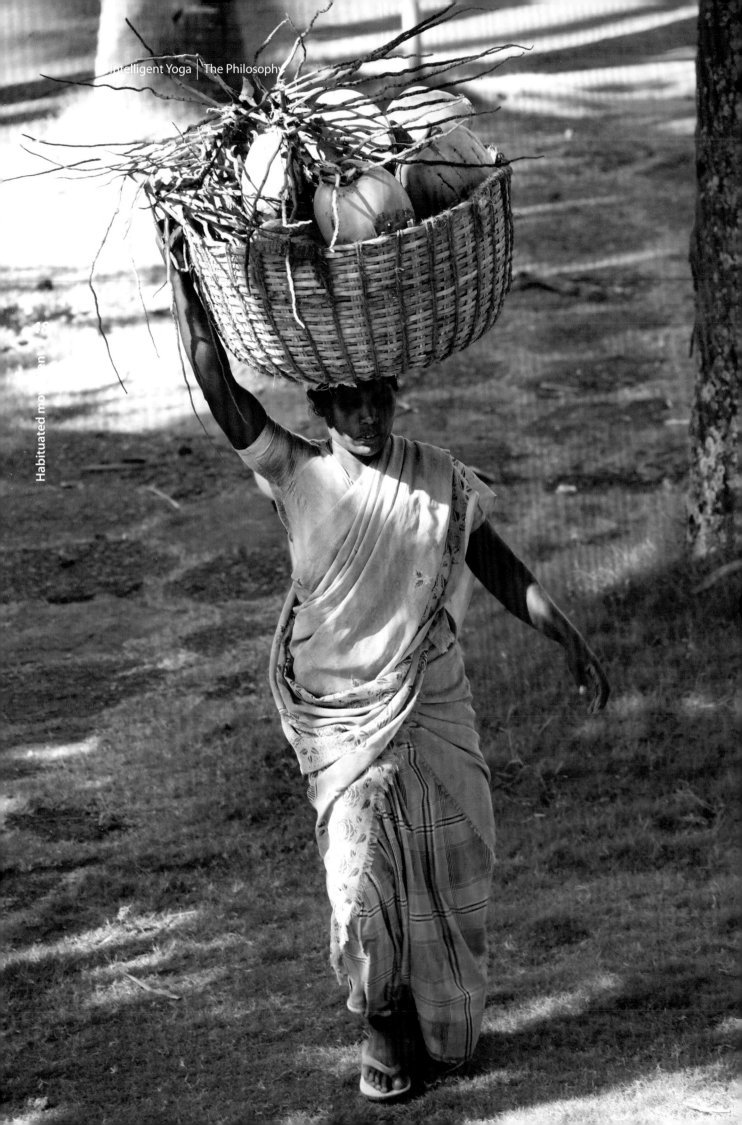

CHAPTER FIVE

Habituated movement

In order to survive successfully in a changing world we learn to habituate certain activities. Anything we do repetitively will almost inevitably become habituated. Think of a task such as driving; when we start to learn we think very consciously of how to change gear, when to depress the clutch, and how far to turn the steering wheel. It is an exhausting mental process and most learners have understandably had enough after about an hour.

After a month or two of regular practice however the muscles of the arm and trunk have learned the positions of the gear stick and handbrake; the bite on the clutch is felt instinctively and the pressure on the pedals will be "known" by the legs. All this is an example of habituation, learned muscle responses that require little or no thought.

Habituation is a vitally important process which allows us to act speedily while at the same time keeping our conscious brain clear for more pressing activities. Habituation is to the adult what innate motor reflexes are to the neonate: an efficient means of organising repetitive muscular patterns of movement.

Human beings have the tendency to habituate both appropriate and non-appropriate muscular patterns. Because it is habitual and therefore sub-conscious, we are not aware of the tensions these muscles impose on us, even though it may be obvious to an observer.

My father would always tighten his jaw muscles when he was anxious or irritated. The whole family could read the warning signs but he was oblivious to them, even though they almost certainly contributed to the migraines he regularly suffered.

Nearly all of us have our own habitual tensions and many books have been written about tension patterns and the stress they conceal or reveal. Whatever the pattern, its consequence is to tighten the outer muscular container, damping down inner rhythms and smothering the life pulsations of the body's core.

Whatever patterns we develop there will be consequences. Tension in the neck, jaw and shoulders may predispose us towards headaches. Tension in the diaphragm and belly may lead to digestive problems, while tension in the feet may result in foot problems in later life.

These tensions exist as a result of how we cope and adapt to our environment. If they cause us problems, yoga can be a wonderful way of addressing them. Yoga deals with the big patterned movements of the body – flexion, extension, side-bending and rotation. It is in these kind of movements that our habits are embedded. For example, we move towards back bending and find ourselves doing it all from the lower back, or we move into flexion and do it all from the upper back, or we rotate and do it all

RIGHT
Supporting
muscle
contractions
'learn' the level
of tension
necessary to
perform a task

from the neck. Think of how you reverse your car.

Through the practice of yoga we are able to address these habits of movement. We do this by paying close attention to the way we as individuals move into the big patterns. To help us understand how movement is initiated and interpreted in the body it is necessary to have some understanding of the nervous system's control of voluntary movement. Thinking about a movement is done in the cortex, the cognitive part of the brain. Muscular movement is initiated in the motor cortex, the cognitive part of the brain that deals with movement. Nerves run from the motor cortex in the brain to every muscle in the body. When you decide to lift an arm a message passes from the motor cortex down the motor nerves that supply the arm elevator muscles, and the arm lifts.

This is the motor or voluntary system. What we are completely unaware of when we lift an arm are the various concomitant muscular contractions that have to take place to facilitate arm lifting. The scapular, for example, has to be stabilised, as does the spine, to which it is connected.

So although the action of lifting the arm is voluntary much of what takes place at the same time does so seemingly unnoticed. We must "notice" what happens though, at some level, or the action would be impossible; this noticing is achieved via another part of the nervous system, the sensory nervous system.

The sensory nervous system is constantly monitoring the state of tension and stretch that exists in the muscles, tendons and ligaments; it feeds information back to the brain stem and cerebellum. These are primitive parts of the brain that have developed to help organise the body in relation to gravity.

So when we lift an arm, the brain receives information about how the body's relationship to gravity has changed and makes the necessary adjustments to restore equilibrium. This dialogue goes on all the time. We decide what to do, initiate the movement, and a whole series of unconscious supportive measures is carried out unwittingly.

The more we look at any movement, the more we realise that it is actually an orchestration of movement and not any muscle acting alone. Rather it is a series of muscular contractions that ripple through the body to support the desired outcome. Over time these supporting muscle contractions develop "default" settings. They learn the appropriate level of tension necessary to assist in the task they want to perform.

This is all well and good until, as sometimes happens, the default settings go wrong. There are three main reasons why this might happen. The first is environmental. For example, if we sit hunched over a computer day after day the muscles in the back regularly lengthen while the ones in the front shorten. The supporting muscles will play their part in maintaining this unhelpful position. If we practise it enough it will become an acquired skill and every time we sit at the computer our muscles will hunch us up as they have been taught to do.

The second way settings can go wrong is through pain and injury. If we have hurt our neck we may defend ourselves from the pain by adopting a posture that reduces the pain. If the pain persists or recurs, this defended posture adopted to ease it will become well practised, and will eventually be replayed as the normal setting.

Third, and certainly not least, are the emotional responses: as the only voluntary system in the body, the muscular system reflects, inevitably, what is going on in our minds. Unless you are

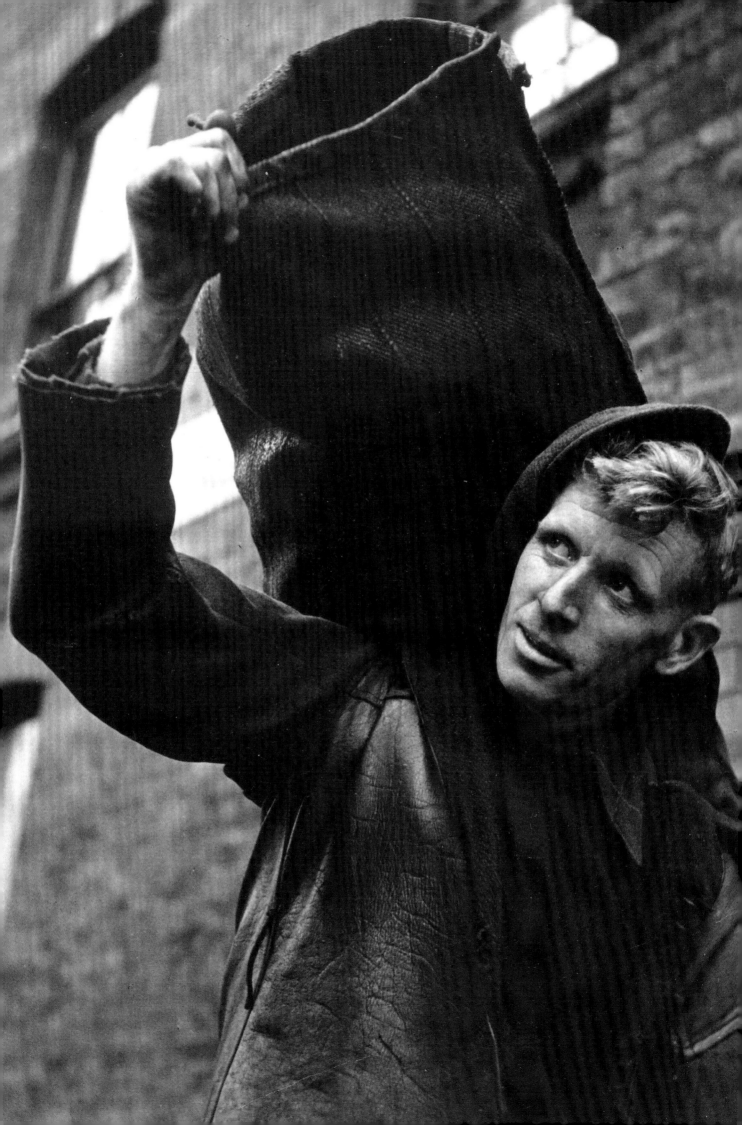

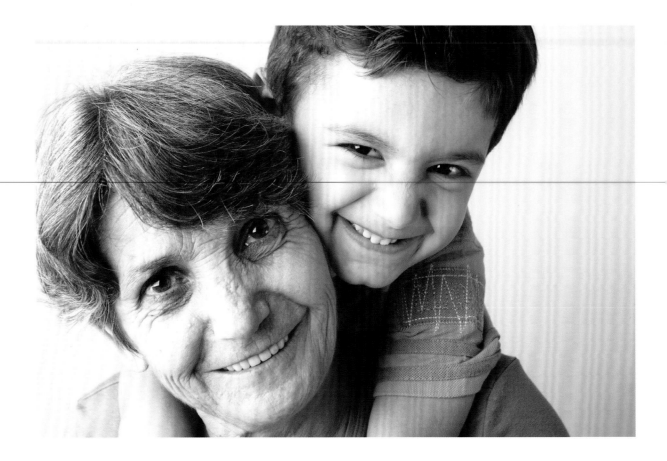

ABOVE
Emotion is
evident in
the faces
and bodies
of those
around us

playing poker or are, for some other reason, with a person who is very good at hiding their feelings, you can see emotion written large into the faces and bodies of all the people around us.

It is a wonderful thing, this individuality expressed in our bodies, the lives we have lived somehow embodied within us. Many of these patterns were "written in" when we were children with little choice in the way we responded to the world.

A child in an uncomfortable world will have to defend himself against the injustices they feel. By the time maturity is reached, these childhood patterns have become deeply embedded in the body, even if no longer consciously sensed.

What is important is that patterns require practise to become embedded and this is equally true for those we want to acquire and those we do not. Take for example a pianist learning a new piece. They will have to learn the spatial and temporal relationships between the notes, the exact pressure required to elicit the correct sound.

This starts as a cortical process, perhaps with frowning; movements have to be repeated

until the desired sequence of notes is achieved. Gradually the cerebellum starts to recognise the feeling of these movements and begins to remember them.

It is tempting to think that the patterns are remembered as a list of instructions stored in the muscles, and all we have to do is remember the list to repeat the pattern again. But this is not the case. Think about writing your signature; written with a biro at a desk, most of the muscles used are in your hand and wrist. Write your signature on a blackboard with chalk, and it is still recognisable, despite having been produced by a different set of muscles (those of the arm and shoulder).

It is obvious when you think about it that it cannot be the motor cortex and the muscles that "remember" patterns. This is an observation backed up by the research quoted in Deane Juhan's book *Job's Body: A Handbook for Bodywork*[8]: "Removal of small parts of the motor cortex that control the muscles normally used for skilled activity does not prevent the monkey from performing the activity. Instead, he automatically uses other muscles in the place of the paralyzed ones to perform the

By the time maturity is reached, childhood patterns have become deeply embedded in the body, even if no longer consciously sensed

same skilled activity… If, on the other hand, we do not tamper with the motor cortex, but instead destroy cell bodies in the sensory cortex which corresponds to the area of muscles, skin, and joint involved in the performance of the original skill, we find something even more arresting; the monkey loses all ability to repeat the skill.

"It is not the motor cortex itself that controls the pattern of activity to be accomplished. Instead, the pattern is located in the sensory part of the brain, and the motor system merely 'follows' the pattern."

This makes it clear that learning patterns is done via the feeling centres of the brain and not the command centres. Teaching this in yoga makes a huge difference to the way in which we approach instructions. If we ask students to follow commands, learning will be less effective than if we ask them to pay attention to the feeling of movement.

If we are to change patterns, we first have to unearth the habit that is embedded in our movement – to understand how we move. This is best achieved by exaggerating an action. If we habitually hold the pelvis in an anterior tilt,

this habitual posture will be hidden, or "unfelt". However, if we exaggerate the movement we consciously engage the same muscles, so that now we can feel them.

We then need to open up some other choices for the body, such as posterior tilting and all the positions between posterior and anterior tilting, and see how these feel. The more these movements are practised and "felt" the more automatic they become.

Be aware, however, that when we practise a new action it needs to be kept as simple as possible; we must be sure we don't practise it with a furrowed brow, for example, because this too will be remembered by the sensory nervous system and "played back", alongside the desired movement.

A good musician pays close attention to the way he sits or holds his instruments; otherwise poor posture will be a constant accompaniment to his music.

To recap: learning is initially a cortical event that is analysed and thought through; later it becomes patterned in the brain, and is replayed in the way it was written. We must, therefore, ensure we write a good script.

54

An intelligent approach

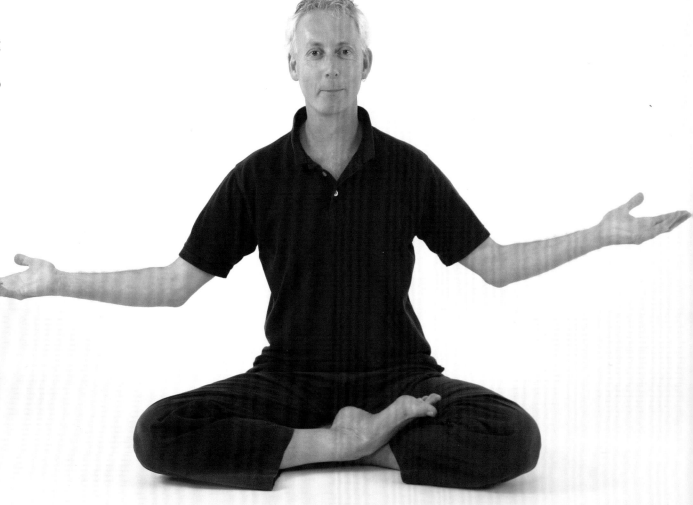

CHAPTER SIX
An intelligent approach

To make the most of our yoga practice, it makes sense to clarify why we practise in the first place. Most people would agree that this is in some way related to a desire to be more comfortable; to feel we inhabit ourselves well. We also need to feel comfortable in our surroundings, and comfortable with other people. Some would choose to take this further and want to feel comfortable with God, or their "spiritual side".

The most important thing about practice is that it should not harm us. This seems an obvious statement but many people hurt themselves doing yoga, and this shouldn't happen. There are several reasons why people hurt themselves while practising yoga. The first of these is ambition. Many yoga postures require great flexibility or strength, and sometimes both. If we attempt to go beyond our capabilities, either because of our own drive or a teacher's over enthusiasm, we can easily come to grief. Overdoing it in yoga can result in pulled muscles, strained ligaments and damaged joints.

Our approach to practice must therefore be an intelligent one; we need to establish our limitations and work within them. These limitations will be different for everyone; some of us are supple, others are stiff. We can all do yoga but we need to select the postures we practise with care. Everyone can start every posture, but

not everyone is able, necessarily, to complete that posture. The skilful yogi will know how far it is useful to go, or indeed take their student, down each particular posture path.

Another reason we can hurt ourselves is because of inattentiveness. Yoga is a powerful tool for change and sometimes demands complex positioning of the body; inattentiveness at such times can cause injury. Ideally, we build up a gradual understanding of the principles of practice, first for the easier postures and later for complex ones.

Sometimes flexible people attempt postures that they don't fully understand. This is often another cause of injury. Being stiff can be a blessing in yoga; understanding often comes first with stiffer people, who tend not to attempt more difficult postures.

The third and perhaps most pernicious reason why people hurt themselves in yoga is when a posture has an inbuilt problem; it is tempting to imagine that postures are inherently safe, because they have been around for thousands of years. Any rough edges would surely have been knocked off by now?

Yet not all the postures are really that old – many of the standing postures date little further than the middle of the 20th century. Also, in guru-led yoga, there is a tendency to stick to tradition without ever questioning it.

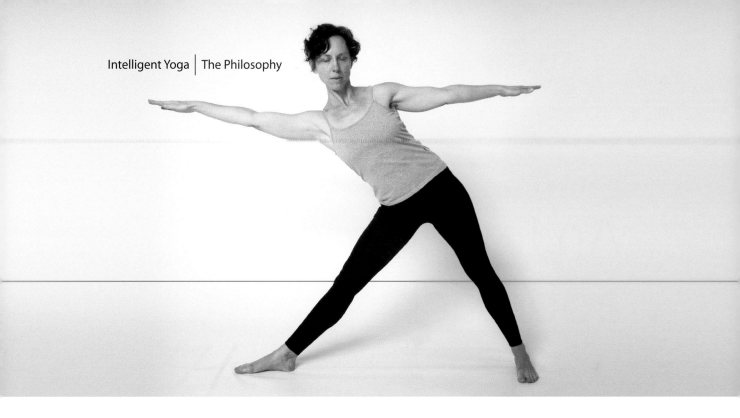

ABOVE
There has been little critical analysis of postures practised in Iyengar yoga

The modern asana tradition

Many of the asanas, or postures, practised today are derived from the teaching of BKS Iyengar, who has done a tremendous amount to develop yoga practice in the West. As a student of Krishnamacharya, the 20th century Indian yogi widely referred to as the father of modern yoga, Iyengar comes from an established and respected line of Indian yoga teachers. It is perhaps because of this, and because of our Western understanding of the traditional guru-pupil relationship in Indian culture, that there has been very little critical analysis of the postures practised in Iyengar yoga – even an unwillingness to change them.

Closer inspection however reveals that far from being ancient yogic practices, there is little evidence that many of the standing poses we practise today date back to before 1935. Film footage of Iyengar and Krishnamacharya demonstrating asana practice in the early 1930s shows many familiar yoga postures, but very few of these are standing poses. It would appear that standing postures were not developed until later, by Krishnamacharya, when he was teaching yoga at the Mysore Palace in southern India. This is described in detail by NE Sjoman in his 1999 book *The Yoga Tradition of the Mysore Palace*[9]. His teachings appear to have been influenced heavily by Western gymnasts who were teaching there at the same time. They also seem to draw strongly on exercises from traditional Indian wrestling.

One can follow a different lineage of asana tradition in Theos Bernard's 1941 book *Hatha Yoga*[14]. Bernard claims to have learnt yoga in an authentic tradition, and demonstrates many poses and practices familiar to the contemporary yogi, particularly those found in the *Hatha Yoga Pradipika*. Here too, a lack of standing postures is conspicuous. More recently, books by Mark Singleton and Elizabeth De Michelis have challenged the view that there is any connection between modern postures and ancient ones. Many other modern systems of body education, such as Feldenkrais, Body-Mind Centering and the Alexander Technique have developed without the albatross of yoga's lineage. They have also had the freedom to develop and evolve in response to new understanding in biomechanics and physiology.

I believe that it Is both legitimate and sensible to look critically at the poses we practise, to reflect on their potential benefits or the harm they may inflict on the practitioner – and to suggest possible improvements.

One of the main intentions of this book is to review the asana tradition, and reappraise it from the standpoint of the human body. This includes, as we have already seen, the effect of gravity on our posture and our breathing.

The importance of gravity

As a species, we've been bipedal for two or three million years. The innate responses we have developed to gravity are reflex and unconscious. The better we can work with them, rather than interfere with them. When considering posture work we need to consider too the likely reflex responses to a position. We must also ensure that a posture is bio-mechanically safe.

Perhaps the most difficult-to-convey aspect of teaching and learning yoga is journey from structure to freedom. It is important to understand the reason for practicing any given posture – what is its point? Remembering, always, that this point may change depending on the intention of the practitioner, and that any posture can offer a number of benefits.

As long as you are clear about what you want from your practice, you have a good chance of being rewarded. But if your practice is unclear and muddled you risk going around in circles and making only limited progress.

Take patterned movements such as extension for example; if we simply practise back bends with no clear idea of from where we should bend and how we should breathe, we will simply bend in the ways that are familiar to our body. We might enjoy the freedom of the movement, but certainly not the back pain that too often accompanies it.

Making the decision to constrain one area of the back when back bending – the lower back, for example – so that we move from a stiffer area (in this case, the upper back) means that the movement becomes more useful and, more importantly, less rooted in old habits.

There may be times however when the freedom of a patterned movement is important, where we don't apply constraint. This is often the case with people who have had chronic pain, and have consequently forgotten how to move freely. The point is that we need to be clear before we start a posture about what we are going to do in order to ensure we achieve the maximum benefit.

Passive and active postures

Postures can be divided into passive and active ones. Passive postures employ gravity, an example being a relaxed forward bend or some of the seated forward bends (if, that is, you have the length in the hamstrings to relax into these bends). Their effect is largely on the connective tissue and muscles of the body. Overstretching or forcing a stretch can destabilise joints if the ligaments are pushed too far.

Because they require little of no muscular effort, one can hold these postures comfortably for as long as it takes for tissues to lengthen, while the muscles rest. They can be useful postures to practise if you are tired or feeling unwell, and are in themselves recuperative.

Active postures are obviously different; they engage the muscular system and therefore the nervous system. These poses will strengthen the muscular system but will also pattern the nervous system. As we practise active poses regularly, the nervous system is programming

RIGHT
In the standing forward bend muscles work to control our descent, and can then become passive

itself to recognise the patterns of movement we use. Passive postures will not do this. A practice comprising solely passive stretches will have little effect on changing one's posture or movement habits.

Sensible yoga practice involves both passive and active components. This can sometimes be contained in one pose; moving slowly into a standing forward bend, for example, requires eccentric activity of the extensor muscles of the body until the full forward bend has been reached. From this point the muscles become quiet and the posture is held by the connective tissue. It can be useful to try and imagine the relationship between the work muscles do, the work the connective tissues do and that done by gravity. Too many anatomy books feature an over-simplification of this relationship particularly when it comes to the pairing of agonist and antagonist, which we will now look at in more detail.

The agonist/antagonist debate

Antagonist means "in opposition". Muscles may be agonist and/or antagonist. The prime mover in any action over a joint might be the agonist, or it might be the force of gravity. Resistance might be provided by the antagonist or it might be provided by gravity.

According to *Gray's Anatomy*: "Prime mover activity is always replaced by gravity when this is appropriate". The only time when gravity is not an issue is when this movement is carried out on the theoretical horizontal plane; that is, sideways movement with no vertical fluctuation. In gravity assisted movements the

agonist moves the body part out of the gravity line, then becomes passive; gravity is then the prime mover. The antagonist is then active, eccentrically contracting to control the speed and rate of movement.

A standing-forward bend, for example, the psoas moves the trunk out of the gravity line and gravity brings the upper body down, while the hamstrings and erector spinae lengthen slowly to control the movement. Once they have reached their limits these muscles "switch off". At this point resistance is provided by the elasticity of the connective tissue.

In gravity resisted movements the agonist remains active, controlling the speed and rate of movement. The agonist is therefore also the prime mover. Gravity provides resistance and the antagonist is passive, yielding to allow movement.

When lifting a leg while standing it is the iliopsoas that does the major part of the lifting in other words the agonist is the prime mover. The hamstring and gluteus maximus yield and gravity provides resistance.

Of course these rules apply in simplistic, body mechanics-related terms, but are always complicated by the pneumatic and hydraulic action of the respiratory mechanism and by the body's visceral support. Movements never function in isolation. It may be useful here to reflect on the mechanisms keeping the body upright, and in so doing resisting gravity. All too often we imagine that our muscles are the only means by which we can support ourselves. This is far from being true, as we will see in the following chapter.

It can be useful to try and imagine the relationship between the work muscles do, the work the connective tissues do and that done by gravity

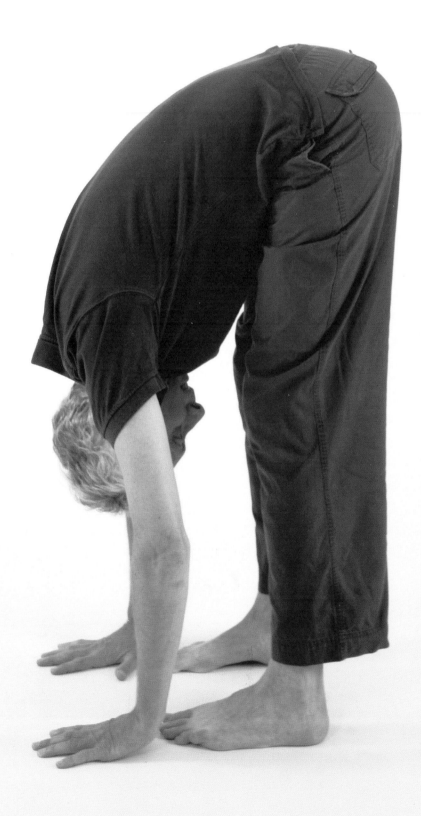

The body's supporting mechanisms

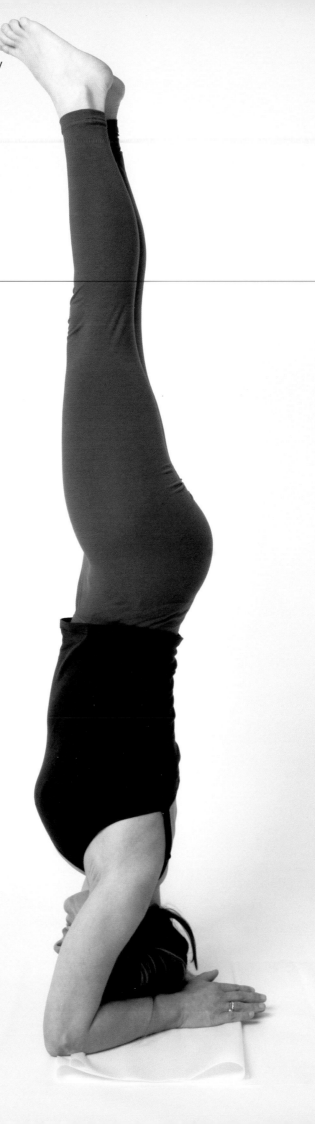

CHAPTER SEVEN
The body's supporting mechansims

Over millennia, the human body has developed sophisticated mechanisms to deal with the relentless pull of gravity. As is true for all living things, energy efficiency is a prime evolutionary advantage and many of the body's gravity addressing mechanisms reduce the effort and, therefore, the energy required for standing and moving.

It is useful to have some knowledge of these mechanisms because improving them will lead to greater ease of movement and reduce the amount of effort we need to complete a task. They include the load-bearing ability of the bones; the activity of the muscular system to support weight and stabilise bones; the elastic forces of connective tissue; tensegrity; the hydrostatic forces of fluids in the body; the hydraulic forces of fluids of the body; and the coordinating activity of the nervous system.

Their relative influence and importance depend on what we are doing. During quiet standing it is tempting to think of the body being supported by the bones. They do after all provide stiffness, and familiar images of the human skeleton nestled at the centre of the body helps reinforce the illusion that the bones on their own support us. Yet take away the body's other supporting structures and what you are left with is a pile of bones.

Human bones have many functions, including providing leverage when muscles act upon them – and in so doing making movement an efficient process. They also transmit forces. When we walk or run the force of the weight of our body is received largely through the skeleton. With a well-organised body these forces will be dissipated evenly through the rigid structure of bones and through the movement of the joints.

Even the rhythm of the breath can be felt moving through the skeletal system, something that would be unlikely if it were bracing to support body weight. While some of our weight is carried by the bones, particularly those of the legs and feet, it is erroneous to think that all our weight is borne by the skeleton alone. Bones, as we have seen, need other mechanisms to hold them in place and to enable them to move.

Muscles generate power and therefore seem well equipped to deal with this. Most of us are aware of the concept of postural or anti-gravity muscles. Yet our muscles comprise an energy intensive system; the more we need them to hold us up the more energy we consume. An energy efficient body will therefore employ as little muscular activity as possible.

Most of the muscles in the body are designed for movement rather than for holding us up. When muscles act over joints and exert a force on bones, efficient movement is made possible. But it is in the interest of the individual that when movement ceases, muscle activity quietens

It helps to think of the human structure as an inverted pendulum with the fixed point being the feet and the greatest sway being at the head

down. In fact, quiet standing uses little more energy than lying down.

Debate rages over which of our muscles are meant to be postural. Some physiologists base their opinion on the amount of "slow-twitch" fibres present within a muscle, believing that a greater preponderance of slow-twitch fibres must exist to support sustained activity.

Others take a bio-mechanical viewpoint, calculating the force required to keep a body from falling and deciding which muscles might provide this force.

More convincing to me are those who study electromyographic activity – the measurable activity of a muscle – despite the fact that this reveals only which muscles are working, and not those which are the most useful.

It helps to think of the human structure as an inverted pendulum with the fixed point being the feet and the greatest sway being at the head. One would expect then to find that balance is maintained by long muscles reaching upwards from the base, which indeed seems to be what happens.

But as Basmajain and De Luca point out in their book *Muscles Alive*[10], it is not the continued activity of these muscles that keeps us upright, but rather phasic activity which takes account of the almost imperceptible sway we all have when standing. Muscles only become active when we sway too far; the elasticity of the tendons of the feet and legs tether the body,

thus reducing muscular activity.

However, research has shown that the soleus muscle in the calf is the most actively engaged muscle when we stand, and therefore has perhaps the best claim to be a true postural muscle. The tibialis anterior at the front of the calf and gastrocnemius at the back exhibit the kind of intermittent activity one might expect to counteract sway.

Activity in both sets of muscles increases significantly when we walk or stand on our toes or when we wear high heels.

We see a similar pattern In the muscles of the thigh as those exhibited in the muscles of the lower leg; phasic activity that compensates for postural sway. There is certainly no necessity for continued action of the thigh muscles to maintain upright standing.

Interestingly one muscle of the hip shows continuous activity, and this is the iliopsoas. This is probably to keep the trunk balanced on the legs, while the strong hip ligaments resist hyper extension of the joint.

There is, however, a fair amount of variation between individuals: some people exhibit virtual quiescence in the erector spinae, while others experience considerable activity. In my experience, people with chronic back pain are often over using these muscles. It makes sense then, if one can, to stand with quiet muscles.

We should note that one group of abdominal muscles, the internal obliques, experience

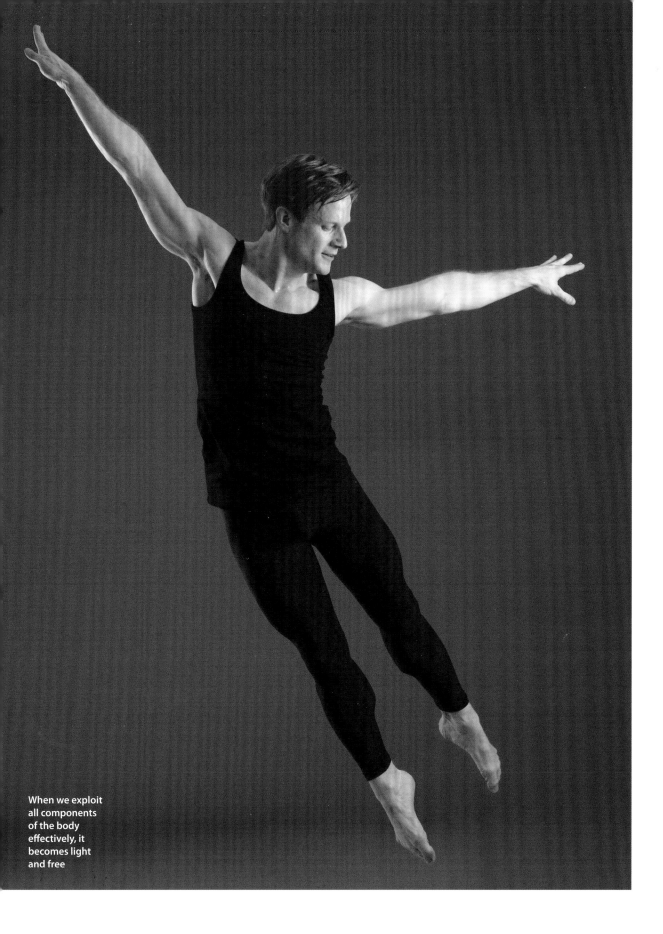

When we exploit all components of the body effectively, it becomes light and free

constant activity when one is standing upright. These muscles almost certainly support the weight of the viscera as they bear down on the pelvic floor and lower abdomen. This is probably also true of the transverse abdominals, but because these are such deep muscles this is difficult to measure.

The head and neck together provide plenty of scope for variations in the ways individuals support themselves, and some activity of the posterior muscles of the neck is necessary to prevent the head from falling forward. Although the upper trapezius could (and in some people does) perform this role, this is neither essential nor desirable. Rather it is more efficient when the deeper neck extensors take on this role, the most useful of these being splenius capitus and cervices .

Recent research on the spine indicates that the very deepest layers of muscles spanning individual vertebra have a local stabilising effect, while the outer muscles are used more for global movement. This suggests that muscular stability works from the inside out; if the inner muscles do their job, the outer muscles can get on with actions rather than supporting the body.

We need to remember, of course, that quiet standing is a rare event and the muscles are in a state of constant interplay with gravity. Whenever we move and gravity needs to be resisted, muscles have to act. The better-organised we are, the less activity is needed.

When you study the musculature of the human body you cannot help but be struck by the abundance of connective tissue. Although not hugely extensible, collagen, the principle protein of connective tissue, does have elastic properties. Indeed in his book *Elastic Properties in Animal Movement*[11], J McNeil Alexander points out that the Romans sometimes made catapults out of horse and camel tendons.

This connective tissue supports the skeleton in a similar way to that in which guy ropes support the frame of a tent. Slight sway will be restrained by a pull on elastic tissue, and in many areas of the body it is this elastic restraint that preserves muscular effort.

Indeed the connective tissue running through the inside of all muscles provides them with a varying degree of elasticity. We often find elastic tension and muscular activity acting harmoniously to provide smooth and easy movement. If we look at the knee for instance, the Achilles tendon and associated muscles join forces with the hamstring tendon to open and straighten the leg. It is not then the job of the quadriceps to keep the legs straight, as we can

see in the diagram on page 65. It is also true that the medial rotation of the femur on the tibia during the final few degrees of straightening create a stable "locking" of the joint, as the articular surfaces share a snugly fitting position.

The sheets of fascia that run alongside the spine provide a kind of posterior guy rope to help resist the body's tendency to bend forward; in so doing, they relieve the erector spinae of some of their work.

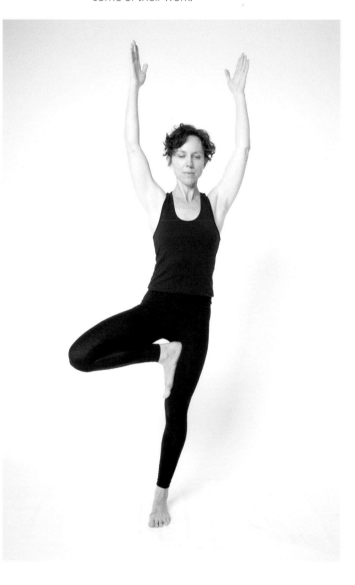

In the foot, it is the spring ligaments that support the arch, not the intrinsic muscles, which become active only once we move.

In breathing, the elastic recoil of the lungs is partly responsible for the contraction of the thorax during exhalation. So to some extent we are being drawn in from the inside when we breathe out.

In addition to its guy rope effect on the body, the elasticity of connective tissue helps absorb shock in movement, acting as a spring when we run and reducing enormously the energy required for locomotion.

The concept of tensegrity was developed by architect Buckminster-Fuller in the 1950s and '60s, when he built the first geodesic domes. The idea that the musculoskeletal system is a tensegrity structure has some appeal, because if the body can be modelled in such a way, it would provide an environment where compressive forces through joints could be counteracted by inherent tensional forces.

Fluids, when contained by the body's muscles and connective tissue, also create pressure, and this pressure provides a very effective response to gravity, in fact hydrostatic pressure is one of the only natural responses to gravity.

Human beings are using all the aforementioned supporting mechanisms all of the time. Emphasis shifts from one system to another as the body moves. Bones, elasticity and fluid support require little muscular input. In fact, we often have to reduce muscular effort to make more effective use of these systems. Yet because the muscular system is the only one we can knowingly engage, many of us over use and exhaust what is actually the most compliant of systems. The intelligent practise of yoga can help mitigate such over use, as I explain later in the posture section of this book.

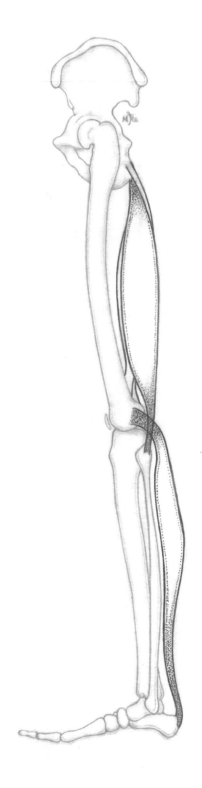

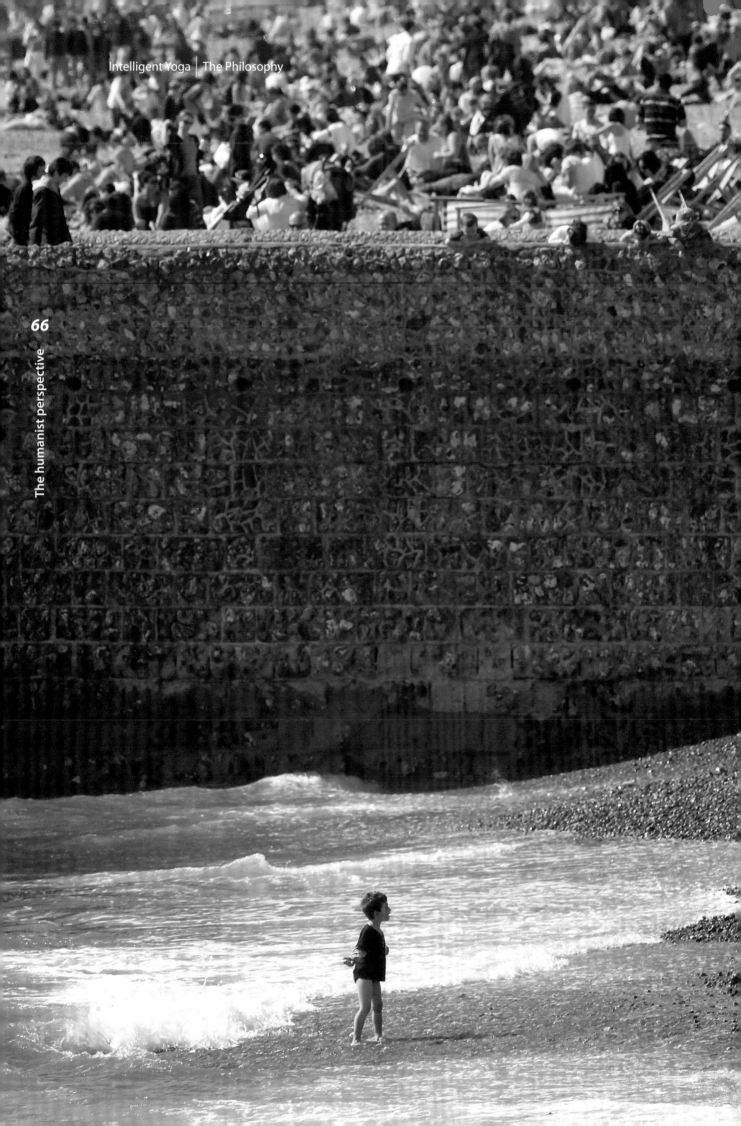

66

The humanist perspective

CHAPTER EIGHT

The humanist perspective

Yoga holds a unique place in the exploration of the human condition. On the one hand it can draw on a rich historical heritage, while on the other, the direct experience of the practitioner keeps it forever in the present.

Having a history is useful, as I pointed out in the opening chapter of this book. It gives context to the modern practice, or at least it has the potential to do so. There is also a danger though that we become led by our history and instead of seeking to build on the understandings of those who have gone before, we conform our experience to fit what we have been led to expect. This, I would argue, is the biggest challenge to the modern yogi.

So what are the understandings of the modern world and how do they fit into yoga? In this chapter I will attempt to outline some of the discoveries and insights that have made an impact on me and enriched my understanding of the human condition.

I've noticed that many people feel discomforted if the metaphysical world is challenged; this sometimes surprises me because the world I see is more complex, exciting and exhilarating than anything I could imagine.

I can understand that this starting point can seem bleak; we are born alone and we die alone, and I'm pretty sure we don't carry on after that.

For me this is the bottom line, and facing up to this reality is the ultimate challenge of being human. I don't want to fabricate any false promises or positions to try and make myself feel better about it. Rather I want to develop the qualities that enable me to live a life with this knowledge and without fear.

I think this recognition is essential because understanding the concept of being alone is an important one, and probably the most misunderstood. The reality is that human beings are never truly isolated.

Without relationships we fail to thrive. Very young children will die without human contact even when they are fed and watered. A slightly older child will suffer brain damage if human contact is removed or reduced to subsistence levels. Throughout our lives the quality of the relationships we form impacts on our state of well-being.

We are a social species and we thrive in communities. Being separated from our fellow humans causes us to suffer. To isolate someone is one of the worst punishments we can inflict on them, and yet strangely we often isolate ourselves.

Loneliness is the discomforting feeling that arises when our relationships are not up to the mark. We need to heed this feeling as our feelings are our primary means of self-regulation. It is also evident that different people have differing

The humanist perspective

needs for social contact. John Cacioppo in his book *Loneliness: Human Nature and the Need for Social Connection*[12] makes the point clearly that some people need a lot of social contact, others less, but it is a very unusual person who thrives in isolation. Being a hermit is almost certainly not the right aspiration for good human health, even if most of us feel the need to be alone from time to time.

We stop "aloneness" becoming loneliness through our ability to form relationships. The skill with which we do this will go a very long way in determining whether our lives are happy or not. It is not too difficult to extrapolate from this that moral frameworks evolve out of social frameworks. In our search for better relationships and the avoidance of isolation we need to look after those who would look after us – we'll scratch their back if they scratch ours.

As societies grow in complexity so do our skills in social interaction. Researchers estimate that as much as 40% of our brain is dedicated to reading the nuances of other people's actions and expressions. It is this socialisation that has driven the expanding size of our brains.

You may ask what has this got to do with yoga, but I think it has everything to do with yoga. Our yoga practice, if performed intelligently, is a self exploration. We learn about the way in which we inhabit our bodies. We learn about muscular habits and patterns that we have laid down in our life and we start to find out what these patterns mean.

Abraham Lincoln famously said that by the time you are 40 you have the face you deserve. To some extent our bodies are "set" in a similar way, although I would not use the word "deserve". Rather, our bodies represent the lives we have lived thus far, our history.

Many of the habits in our nervous systems,

habits exhibited by our muscles, reflect the struggles we have encountered and survived as children. These are the defences and bracings we have needed to get through life. We shut down difficult feelings by holding ourselves in a particular way, in an attempt to make ourselves feel safe.

Our diaphragm, shoulders and hip flexors all play major roles in the containment of feelings, but any muscles can participate. This is particularly true when we try to hide our discomfort. The muscular "disguises" we wear in order to avoid revealing our real feelings eventually become familiar and part of us.

Emotional and physical habits get played out over and over again in everyday life and often bring us discomfort or pain. Therapists might be able to help with the identification of our physical and emotional problems but the real work starts when we start to reflect on our habits and patterns, to discover ourselves and slowly strip away a mantle we no longer need.

Once we manage to remove our unnecessary reflex responses to life we discover that we have choice in the way we respond; instead of doing what we've always done we can do something different.

As other options appear, we become freer; we are better off than if we plod along a reflex pathway that is self confining.

It is not easy to move away from old, ingrained ways of being, but it starts in yoga by the gradual capacity to pay attention. Initially this might be simply how we organise the body in space, noticing for example if our feet are parallel. It can soon develop into an awareness of muscular movement pattern, of how we deal with the breath, or even how we respond to a certain person, who perhaps makes us feel defensive.

RIGHT
Neglect in early life can have profound implications later

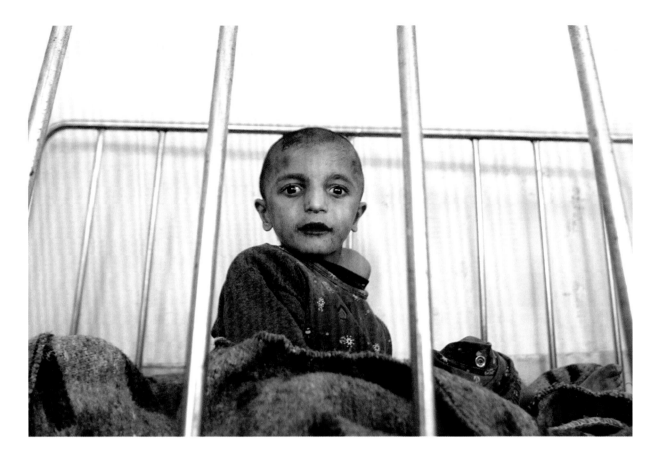

Slowly we can find out more about ourselves, and by doing so become better able to choose our responses. This, I think, defines maturity. As we get older and lose the spring of youth, the sense of being a more complete person is good compensation. Friendships can broaden and deepen, and our capacity to love – the pinnacle of human achievement – becomes greater. And so the life we live, the only life we have, becomes richer and more nourishing.

Those people who are interested in this kind of personal journey can suffer a fair amount of discomfort on the way, just as taking off familiar old clothes can leave us feeling vulnerable or bereft. But as we put better strategies in place, our life can take on new and rewarding depth.

Knowing where our difficulties start is intriguing. Emerging research in neuroscience suggests, perhaps unsurprisingly, that these problems start to develop early in our life, in the context of our relationship with our parents. A wonderfully revealing book written by Sue Gerhardt called *Why Love Matters: How Affection Shapes a Baby's Brain*[13] shows the effects of parental love on brain development.

Our current understanding goes something like this: When a baby is born it is completely unable to deal or regulate its feelings. When discomfort develops in a child up to the age of about three, the child experiences stress. However, we can now measure levels of stress in babies by swabbing their mouth and measuring their cortisol levels. As Gerhardt asserts: "Human babies are born with the expectation of having stress managed for them. They tend to have low levels of cortisol in the first few months, as long as caring adults maintain their equilibrium through touch, stroking, feeding and rocking. But their immature systems are also very unstable and reactive; they can be plunged into very high cortisol levels if there is no one to respond to them. Babies cannot manage their own cortisol".

She goes on to note that stress in infancy, such as consistently being ignored when you cry, is particularly hazardous because high levels of cortisol in the early months of life can also affect the development of other neurotransmitter systems whose pathways are still being established.

"They are still immature and are not fully developed even by weaning time. Babies of

A *child unable to regulate his or her feelings will grow into an adult (and possibly parent) who struggles with those same feelings*

The humanist perspective

withdrawn mothers, for example have lower epinephrine, norepinephrine and dopamine than other babies. When stressed, these various biochemical systems may become skewed in ways that make it more difficult for the individual to regulate his or her feelings later in life."

For many parents the information revealed in Gerhardt's book makes for uncomfortable reading. I for one was brought up in a time when being left to cry was considered to be good for a baby's lungs. Mothers were told to feed their babies every four hours.

We are now starting to learn that these ideas are wrong, they may have been well meant but they cause suffering. On reflection, we can see too that such approaches are counter-intuitive; mothers are "wired" to respond to a crying baby, not to ignore it.

The reason some parents manage better than others almost certainly has something to do with their own childhood, and how well regulated they were as babies. A child unable to regulate his or her feelings will grow into an adult (and possibly parent) who struggles with those same feelings. They may, for example, find it almost impossible to engage with their own baby's emotions in a productive and responsive way, and so the cycle continues.

I feel now that we are approaching a time when this negative cycle can be broken, and we may eventually be able to produce generations of children who are "in touch" with their feelings, and so do not have to look for other people or belief systems to do the regulating for them.

Gerhardt believes that the problems individuals encounter in adult relationships are often rooted in the poorly developed relationship they had with their parents as children.

Erich Fromm touches on this, with respect to

Christianity, in his book *The Art of Loving*[14].

Fromm believes that our relationship to God mirrors our relationship to our parents, particularly the one we have to our father. The Old Testament's God is a somewhat severe, domineering father figure who demands to be obeyed. In the New Testament though, through the teachings of Jesus, we learn the qualities that we need to become a good member of society, qualities such as compassion, love and forgiveness. Nevertheless, we are still dependent on God's mercy for our salvation.

Fromm goes on to argue that we eventually embody those qualities of God which we find valuable, in the same way that we take the lessons from our parents in order to move from childhood into adulthood. In the end we have to survive without our parents and learn to make judgements on our own. In the same way, says Fromm, we can leave God behind because in a sense we take in the teaching we value and become our own moral guardian. This is the final act of self responsibility, of growing up.

A similar theme was developed by the Bishop of Woolwich, John Robinson, in 1963. He argued in his ground-breaking book *Honest to God*[15], that God was not "out there", but within each of us. He described God as the "ground of our being" and encouraged "depth" in people's lives.

Although Fromm was a humanist and Robinson a Christian, I am struck by how similar their views are, with both emphasising relationships as a route to a meaningful life, and embracing love as the summit of life's journey.

Yet our relationship to God or our dependence on metaphysical belief systems can be as intransigent as our relationships to other people. It is as if we need them to fill a space our parents could not fill.

Richard Dawkins, in his book *The God*

Delusion[15], adds another strand to the view that we are led by our history into our relationships with God or powerful people. Here, however, it is not the history of the individual, but rather the history of the species. Dawkins points out that, from an evolutionary point of view, it makes a great deal of sense to believe what authority figures are telling us.

No other species on the planet has such a long period of parental dependency as that of humans. For several years we need adult members of the society to help us survive. If an older person says to a child in an authoritative voice "don't play with snakes", the child will tend to obey; evolution will weed out the rashly experimental child.

Poke it and see is not a good survival strategy where snakes are concerned. It is seemingly inbred in humans to do what authority figures tell us. And if we have been psychologically primed in childhood to find a missing parent, and a charismatic guru or religious teacher comes along, our past can then drive us into a predictable relationship with this new parent figure.

There are of course many shades of grey in the way the past drives our present. We all know that feeling of repeating old mistakes over and over again or, in a body sense, getting that same headache, stomach ache or backache in the same circumstances. It is clear that in some way our history has set us up for these patterns of behaviour, and that they are very difficult to resist. Many people have made a lot of money playing on this knowledge. So many self-help books tell us that living in the present will solve

BELOW
Our belief systems can be as intransigent as our relationships with each other

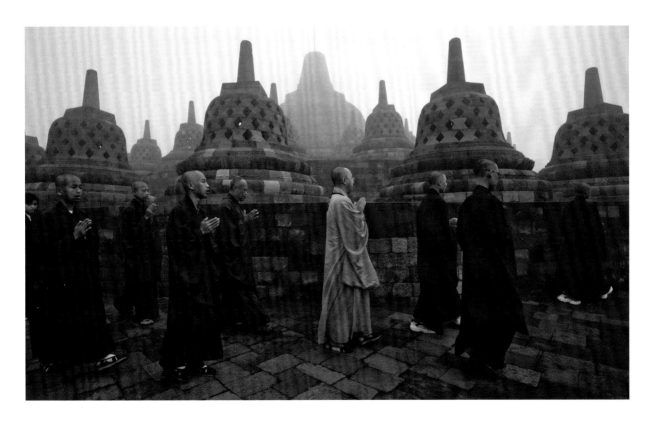

The humanist perspective

our problems. To some extent they are correct; if you can free yourself of your past you free yourself of your patterning, but one cannot simply will this to happen.

So how can yoga help? Neurobiologist Antonio Damasio is one of the world's leading researchers into consciousness and the emergence of feelings and emotions. He argues, in his book *The Feeling of What Happens: Body and Emotion in the Making of Conciousness*[17] that consciousness arrives out of a pre-set condition he calls "the proto self". This, it seems, is a kind of default condition of the human organism, one that is mapped in the lower centres of the brain.

It is important to recognise that we are not conscious of the proto self, but it is the foundation on which all consciousness rests. The next level of consciousness arises when any part of our sensory nervous system is activated. Any input creates a change in the proto self, which responds to all stimuli.

It is the change or modification of the proto self which makes us aware we exist; it seems to be that we know we have a self because we are constantly stimulating the proto self with a stream of sensory input. This input may be external, a sound or smell, or it may be internal, such as thirst or tension. There is never a waking moment when the proto self is not being modified, and so we are constantly aware of our existence. When we sleep and have no input we do not know we exist.

Damasio calls this level of consciousness the "core self". It provides, he argues, the basis for the next level of consciousness, "the autobiographical self". We are all familiar with our autobiographical self, the memories we recall, what we know about ourselves that represent us.

However, memories are distinct from

feelings and feelings, says Damasio, and are the substrate for emotions: "Punishment causes organisms to close themselves in, freezing and withdrawing from their surroundings. Reward causes organisms to open themselves up and out towards their environment, approaching it, searching it, and by doing so increasing both their opportunity for survival and their vulnerability. This fundamental duality is apparent in a creature as simple as a sea anemone. Its organism, devoid of brain and equipped only with a simple nervous system is little more than a gut with two openings, animated by two sets of muscles, some circular others lengthwise. The

BELOW
Opening up is good for the sea anemone

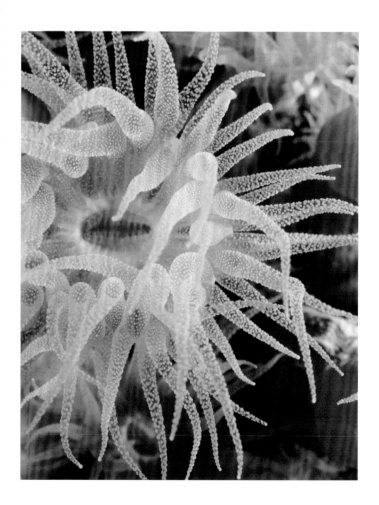

circumstances surrounding the sea anemone determine what its entire organism does: open up to the world like a blossoming flower— at which point water and nutrients enter its body and supply it with energy—or close itself in a contracted flat pack, small, withdrawn, nearly imperceptible to others. The essence of joy and sadness, of approach and avoidance, of vulnerability and safety, are as apparent in this simple dichotomy of brainless behaviour as they are in the mercurial emotional changes of a child at play."

There is a peculiar division that Damasio makes with regard to feelings and emotions. He says that emotions precede feelings, that our response to events occurs before the feelings arise. In fact, he argues, it is the response that causes the feelings. So when something joyful occurs, we respond; we smile, we breathe differently, we relax our shoulders and this causes the feeling of joy.

This may seem surprising, but it is supported by evidence from patients suffering "locked-in syndrome", a condition where only one's eyeballs and eyelids can move. It sounds terrifying. To be fully conscious but trapped in one's body is unimaginably awful. However, it appears that those who suffer this condition have no strong emotional response to their situation. The reason for this is, apparently, that they are unable to make the physiological response to their situation which would otherwise trigger feeling.

It is often said that it is hard to be sad if you put on a smile. It is harder still if you normalise your breathing and adopt a relaxed body posture. Such experiments reveal an intimate relationship between how we feel and the state of our body. It is not a big leap of reasoning to recognise that our habitual patterns of muscular

tension will be associated with habitual patterns of feeling and thinking; it is very difficult to free ourselves from repeating cycles of discomfort – emotional or physical – if we carry our past around in unrecognised muscular patterns.

Internally, all kinds of homeostatic mechanisms ensure that our bodies continue to function. Emotions are our external regulators and we have developed a rich set of these to regulate the relationships that exist in social groups. In more primitive social structures, such as those of apes and monkeys, emotions are probably less sophisticated than those of human beings, but it is easy to see how displays of emotion keep the groups in some sort of order. Mutual fear of predators encourages cooperative feelings, anger and fear establish pecking orders and so on. Any individual ignoring the signals risks violence from stronger males, or expulsion from the group.

Ignoring powerful feelings for too long can, it seems, throw out the feedback mechanisms for our internal regulators. Cortisol levels rise and the risk of illness is increased. Equilibrium – and good health – demands that we respond to feelings and emotions.

Identifying a feeling or emotion before acting upon it appropriately is not as easy as it seems. Many feelings are vague, held as they are by patterns of responding that originate deep in our individual self. Commonly we have emotional "default" settings – we might be angry, ebullient, or melancholic people – but with no particular remembered event to cause such feelings.

In such people, small triggers might initiate a cascade of emotional response. They may, indeed, wonder why they respond so powerfully to certain events. Anyone who has had a relationship with such a person will recognise how difficult in can be; on some level you recognise you are dealing with someone who has lost any choice in how they respond to a particular stimulus. Ultimately, these relationships can become unsatisfactory, lacking as they do spontaneity, depth and surprise.

Through yoga practice we can discover how we tighten our jaw and neck, or fix our diaphragm, and with time we can lose this old and unnecessary tension. Each time we practice without the pattern, the weaker the pattern becomes. And so life becomes simpler.

In the bigger picture this has significant implications. The type of yoga practice I am talking about will lead eventually to greater self knowledge.

Understanding ourselves better leads in turn to greater self trust. There is nothing that interferes with good relationships more than a lack of self trust. When we do not trust ourselves, we have to put our trust in other people, and so our own identity slowly becomes dissipated. We become less attractive to some people, with whom we lose contact, and controlled by others.

Yoga brings into question how we learn, particularly from our teachers; or if we are teachers, how we teach. If we are interested in developing "whole" people, people who can trust themselves and make intelligent choices in life, we need to make sure the conditions are right to bring about such an outcome. We need to consider how we establish an environment where self trust develops.

Learning environments must feel safe. Students need to be able to ask questions without feeling intimidated. Although yoga classes require introspection and peacefulness they are also likely to provoke questioning. Discussion and debate engages people in a way that "top-down" teaching cannot; it breaks

down dogma and reduces the tendency for any "teacher worship" to develop. It also fosters social interaction, something that can be helpful in yoga and life generally.

The larger part of this book explains the anatomy and physiology relevant to yoga practice. I have argued that we need some understanding of the bio-mechanics of the body in order to avoid injury and I try to explain that the breath needs to be responsive rather than controlled. I explain too that some ways of engaging with the body are better than others. I hope I express these points in a way that readers can follow, yet I welcome disagreement and debate.

Not all yoga is like this. There is a long-standing tradition in yoga that wisdom is passed down from guru to student, and because much of yoga's history includes mysticism, there has long been a tendency for obscuring knowledge.

The serious yoga student will, at some point, have to make a decision about belief; whether to abandon one's rational view of the world to pursue one that makes some big promises, a world where suffering can be transcended, where even death may be an illusion.

In many cases this involves surrendering to a guru. This contrasts starkly with self trust and the idea of developing choice and reason. In fact, belief and reason are very different and can lead us in very different directions.

I can understand the relief that surrendering to a belief might bring, but it has a cost – the ability to question and to be open to new ideas. Belief systems cannot stand scrutiny; you buy into the belief or you stand outside it. It is almost impossible to half believe. In belief systems doubt is seen as an obstacle to the truth.

In a system based on rational thought, questions and doubt are assets, providing fuel for debate and discovery. There are times when uncertainty can feel frustrating, but it's one of the conditions of reason; we don't know everything and there is no all-knowing position to be had.

What do we risk losing if we decide not to believe? Not much I think. A reasonable life is not an arid one. Anyone who has experienced the ecstasy of falling in love, the breathtaking beauty of nature, the wonder of music and art, and the curiosity engendered by self exploration, knows that the world can nourish us at the deepest level.

The knowledge that my molecules were formed in stars, and my family line forms an unbroken chain through hundreds of millions of years back to the primordial soup, makes the hairs on the back of my neck stand on end. This and the good friendships we form in life enhance our lives and us as individuals.

The needs of society today are different to those of the society that gave birth to yoga. The idea of rigid duty and unwavering faith in God are no longer as widely appealing as they once were.

Some may ask how we regulate social behaviour and hone our moral and ethical principles if we have moved away from the frameworks that gave life structure in the past. Many books have been written on this subject and this is not one of them. However, I am an optimist and if I believe in anything, I believe in humanity.

The world is shaped by individuals. The more clearly we understand ourselves and our motivations the better chance we have of acting well in the world, and this is really my point.

Yoga can help us to act with understanding and self-awareness, to become mature in the full sense of the word. It is a positive force in a world that struggles to accommodate change.

The world is shaped by individuals. The more clearly we understand ourselves and our motivations the better chance we have of acting well in the world

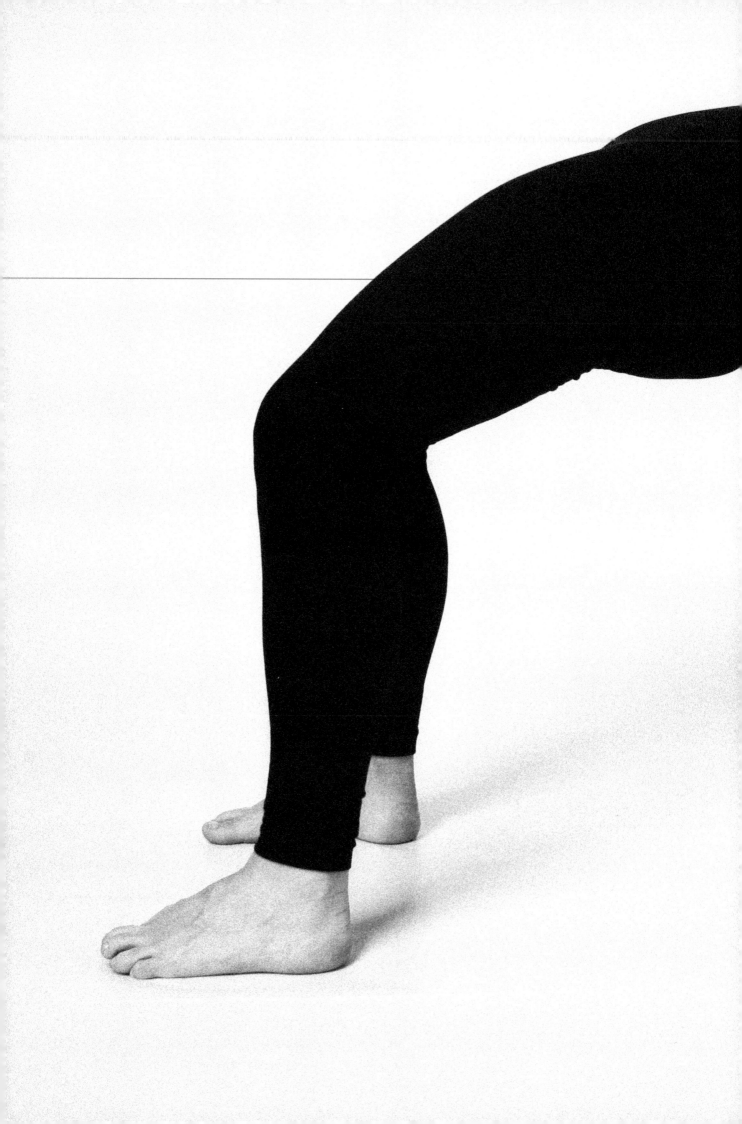

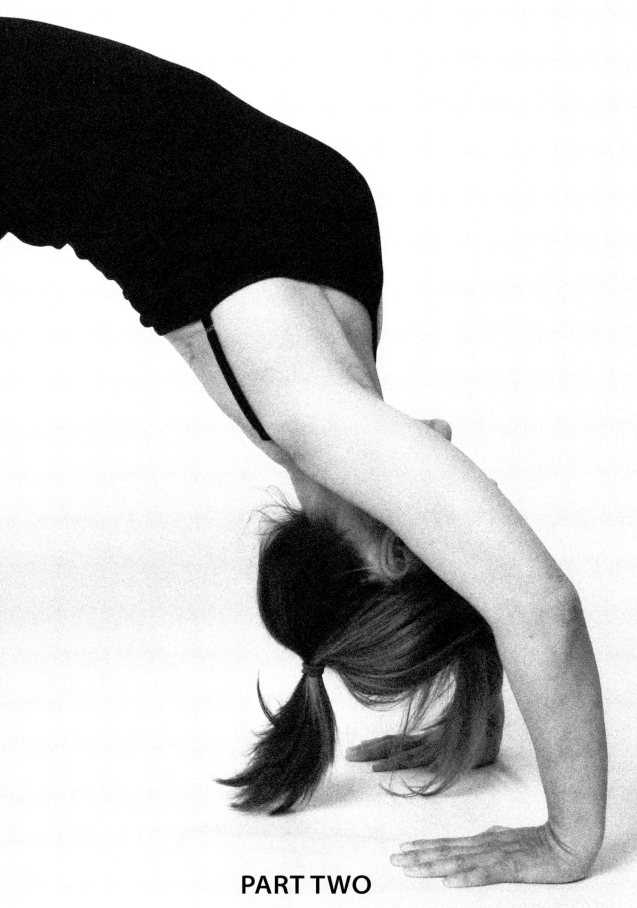

PART TWO
the practice

Grounding and locomotor patterns of movement

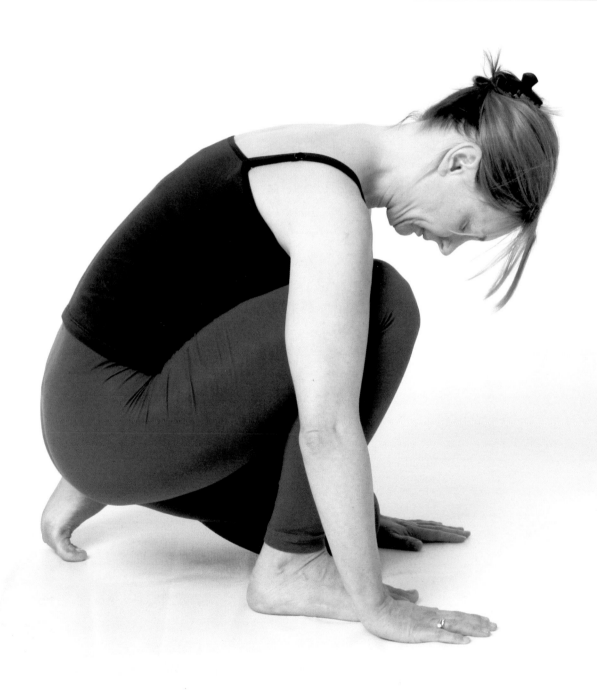

Grounding and the importance of locomotor patterns of movement

The notion of grounding is well known in yoga and other bodywork circles. Its nature can be somewhat elusive; after all, how can one be more or less on the ground? Clearly we cannot become physically heavier or lighter on command, but we can *feel* that we are. Grounding is a subjective experience of feeling more supported by the floor, which gives us a sense of stability and potential for movement.

Physically, things do happen as a result of our capacity to give the weight of our body to the floor without unnecessary interference from muscles. Bones are the only structures in the body that receive and transmit linear forces. When we "find" our bones and allow them to assume a supporting role, muscles can start to relax. It is in the "undoing" of muscles that freedom in the joints is found and with it greater ease in movement.

All posture work should be preceded by a sense of grounding so that we don't carry tension and previously held patterns into our practice. This is a slow but fruitful process, a constant investigation of ways to maintain the integrity of a movement without accumulating tension. It is in this spirit that one should approach all posture work. Here I would like to define tension as unnecessary effort put into an action.

These days, there are a bewildering number of styles of yoga practice, each with its own particular emphasis or history. In the following section on postures I will not be following any tradition or belief.

I will be looking at the postures from the purely human perspective, to the best of my understanding. My intention is to make them as beneficial as possible by explaining the biomechanics involved and, more importantly, our reason for doing them. Unless we have a clear understanding of why we are doing something, it is very difficult to know if we are doing it well or badly.

I have elected wherever possible to use descriptive English titles for postures in preference to more widely used English and Sanskrit names. This is in a bid to avoid ambiguity and to clarify the purpose of the pose.

I would also like to make the point that the following text is not a collection of rules; rather these are principles that can inform one's yoga practice. Rules can lead to dogma; they can dull one's capacity to think. The less we understand, the more hidebound we are by rules. A principle, on the other hand, can deepen one's understanding.

It is important not to try to imitate these postures too literally, but to see them as inadequate representations, or static images, of expansion, contraction, and motion – of living patterns of movement.

We have inherited from our evolutionary ancestors some deeply rooted patterns of movement, which are expressed by the way the muscles control the spine. There is a rather pleasing symmetry in the way movement has evolved and the way in which babies develop movement as individuals. This echoes German

Grounding and locomotor patterns of movement

zoologist Ernst Haeckel's theory of biogenetic law; that ontogeny (the development of the individual) recapitulates phylogeny (the evolutionary history of a species).

The movements displayed by all mobile life forms have their origins in the pulsations of the invertebrates. The first serious attempts at locomotion developed with muscles acting on a skeleton. In fish, this was through the side-bending movements of the spine, controlled by long lateral and intercostal muscles. In infants, the first locomotor reflex we see is the Galant reflex, which initiates side-bending when the baby's side is touched.

When fish left the oceans and pulled themselves on to the land, they evolved into low slung reptiles. Side-bending was still the preferred method of movement – fins became legs, acting at the apex of the side-bending curve increasing the leverage of side-bending propulsion.

The intercostal muscles in lizards act as both respiratory muscles and locomotor muscles for side-bending. This is problematic for the lizard, for running and breathing cannot be accomplished at the same time; running has to be done in short bursts with resting periods in which the lizard can catch its breath.

Serge Gracovetsky, author of *The Spinal Engine*[18], makes the point that when rotation is brought into the side-bending spine, extension is an inevitable consequence. Back-bending almost certainly developed as a result of the early lizards having to twist their way over obstacles in their path.

In mammals, the diaphragm seems to have evolved with the change in position of the legs. As legs moved from the sides to underneath the body, side-bending became less useful as a means of locomotion, and the ribs remained freer for breathing.

Longer legs enabled early animals to move more easily over objects, and the up and down movements of the spine developed more. The diaphragm and soft belly developed firstly to enable respiration and movement to take place at the same time, and secondly to allow greater

BELOW
There is an interesting symmetry between the developmental movements of the child and and those that unfolded in our evolutionary history

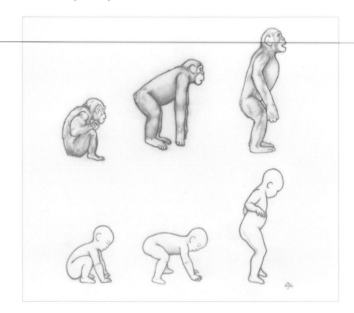

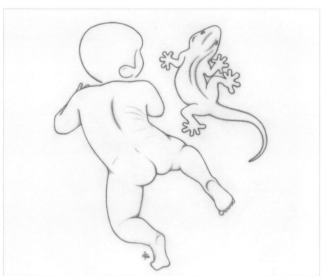

flexion and extension of the body – something necessary for swift movement on land.

Think of the running cheetah, how its body folds as its feet move together, and extends as the legs reach away from each other. This flexion and extension movement of the spine is seen in the tonic extensor reflex and the flexion response of the young baby.

The rotator patterns of bipedal man can also be seen in the rotation motor patterns of the baby when they first start to roll over.

Patterns from our evolutionary history and our own individual history contribute to easy movement. Movement educators such as Moshe Feldenkrais and Bonnie Bainbridge Cohen, and researchers such as Gracovetsky, have long argued that the better the body understands these primary movements, the better organised we tend to become.

It is also worth emphasising that these movements, when distributed well through the body, are safe. They are the movements the body has evolved for, movements the body has grown to accommodate.

I am, therefore, presenting the postures in the following order: side-bending postures, extension postures, flexion postures and rotation postures. I will also examine some of the so-called "classical" postures, which, to my mind, are bio-mechanically unsound. This is not as a criticism, but rather as an attempt to improve the safety and effectiveness of posture practice.

Before any posture is attempted it is worthwhile to quieten yourself as much as possible, to feel steady and relaxed. Then, as an intended movement is developed, you can attempt to sense the quality of the movement you make.

Ask yourself whether you are bringing more effort than is required. Are you adding anything unnecessary to the movement? Are you anticipating the end of the movement? Or are you really trying to sense how you feel, moment by moment, throughout the movement?

In patterns of movement, it is the clarity of the movement that is important and not the amount. Thus, patterned side bends might be quite small movements, but movements undertaken with a lot of attention. The aim is to teach the neuromuscular system to perfect a movement; stretches don't teach the nervous system anything, it is only when the muscles of a patterned movement are asked to act that learning can take place.

Our habits are bound to our patterned movements, so we need to teach ourselves how to move without bringing our history with us. It is very common to see people substituting a more familiar movement for the one requested. Someone whose side-bending is not clear in their body, for example, might when side-bending on all fours introduce side-shifting and flexion of the hips, and rotation of the neck.

When patterned movements are not clear, movement in life can look clumsy and lack grace. It is important that we spend some of our yoga practice addressing how we deal with patterns.

We may simply feel stiff and tight and want to stretch a muscle to relieve it of tension. As our practice develops however this aspect of yoga may become less important; we may have become flexible enough, and now want to improve the way we engage with our body.

When we are clear about what we want we can practise more usefully.

BELOW
The running cheetah displays both flexion and extension in its spine

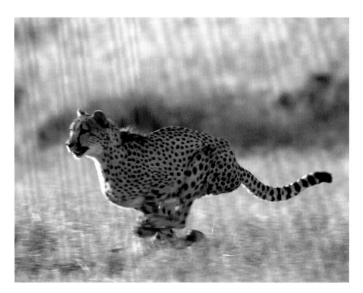

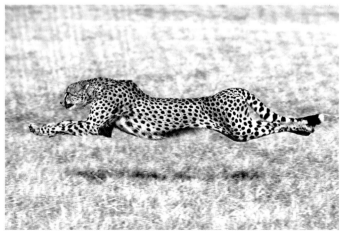

Side bends – the origins of locomotion

All-fours side bend

Here we see side-bending in its purest form; the action is performed by contracting the muscles along the right side, engaging the muscles the baby uses in the Galant reflex, and the fish or salamander in its locomotor movements. These are the erector spinae on the right side, the right-side quadratus lumborum and latissimus dorsi, and the right-side trapezius muscles.

The consequence of activating the right lateral muscles is that the spine will shorten on the right side, the right shoulder will move toward the right hip, and the right hip will move towards the right shoulder.

The muscles on the left side, the antagonists, will lengthen as the agonists on the right side contract. A good relationship between the contracting agonist and the releasing antagonist makes for a useful side-bending movement.

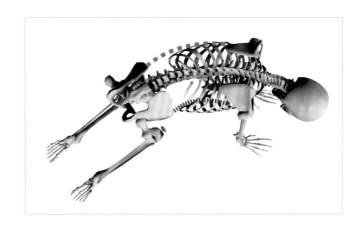

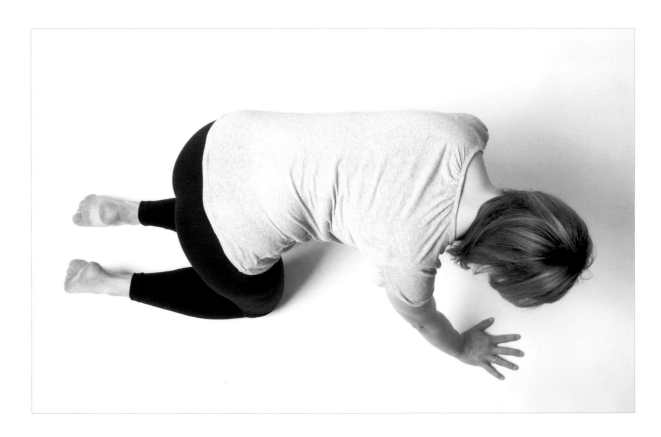

Seated side bend

Parivrtta Janusirsasana

When you look at this pose, often referred to as *Parivrtta Janusirsasana*, you realise it is not a pure side bend; the first component of the posture is rotation, and until reasonable rotation can be achieved it will remain an unsatisfactory posture. The amount of twist in the pose is also related to how wide apart the legs are. The wider the legs, the less rotation is necessary.

However, when there is enough rotation in the thorax, this can be a useful side bend. If we treat the pose as a patterned movement and contract the muscles on the right side, there will be a predictable shortening on this side, accompanied by lengthening on the left side. What is significant here is that the weight will tend to shift on to the left sitting bone.

Side-stretching is different. If you pull with the arm to move the body across the leg, and try to lay the waist along the leg; you risk shearing actions at the lumbosacral joint which can lead to low back problems if practised regularly.

The areas around the sacroiliac joints and the lumbo-sacral joints are designed to be secure; once instability occurs, they are very difficult to stabilise. One of the indications of this type of unhelpful action is that the weight tends to get pulled onto the right sitting bone.

BELOW Sideways reaching movements can cause unhelpful shearing actions at the point indicated by the arrow

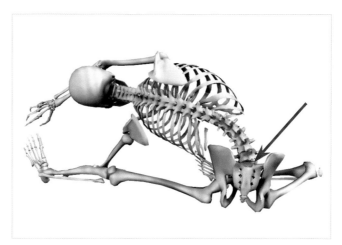

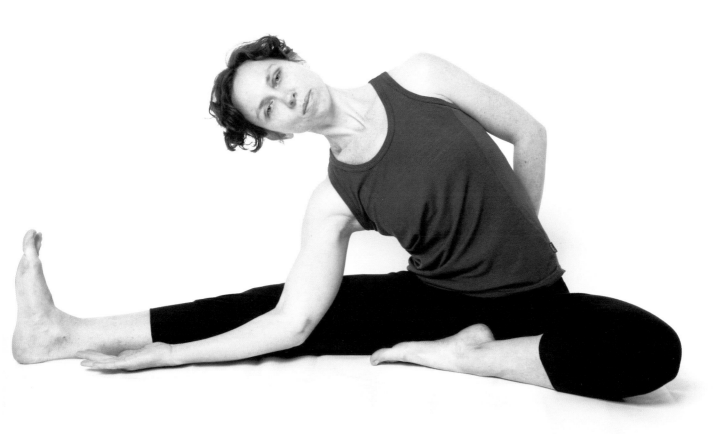

Standing side bends

Gravity is usually the prime mover in these standing side bends. However, if the hips are kept level it is much more of a spinal movement.

One of the main points of working with the major patterns of movement in the body is to notice how well the movement is distributed through the body. In side-bending, one can ask how much is done in the lumbars and thoracic spine, and how much in the neck.

We tend to move from our easy areas. If our lumbar spine is free, we will do most of the work from here. However, if we practise like this all that happens is that we become more mobile in our mobile areas and remain stiff in stiff areas.

If the entire spine "dislikes" side-bending, we may find ourselves moving from the hips instead, as shown below left. We may think we are side-bending more, but we are in reality moving in the ball and socket joints, this stretches the adductor muscles on the side to which we are bending. This is often accompanied by an effort to stretch further, creating similar shearing forces to those accompanying the seated side bend.

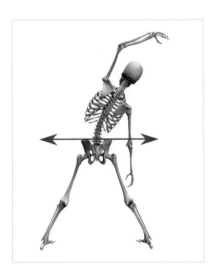

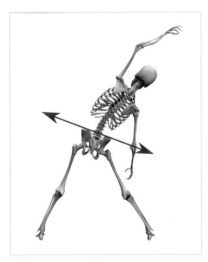

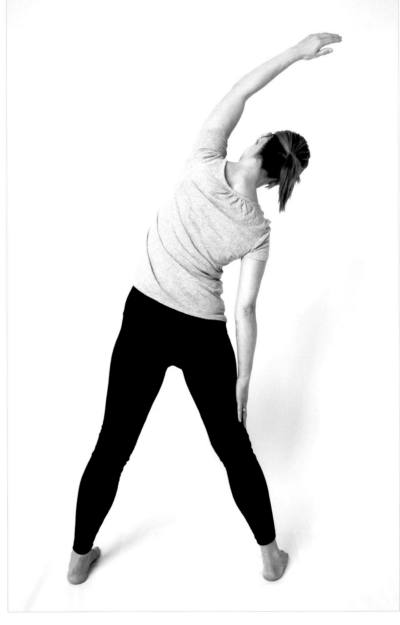

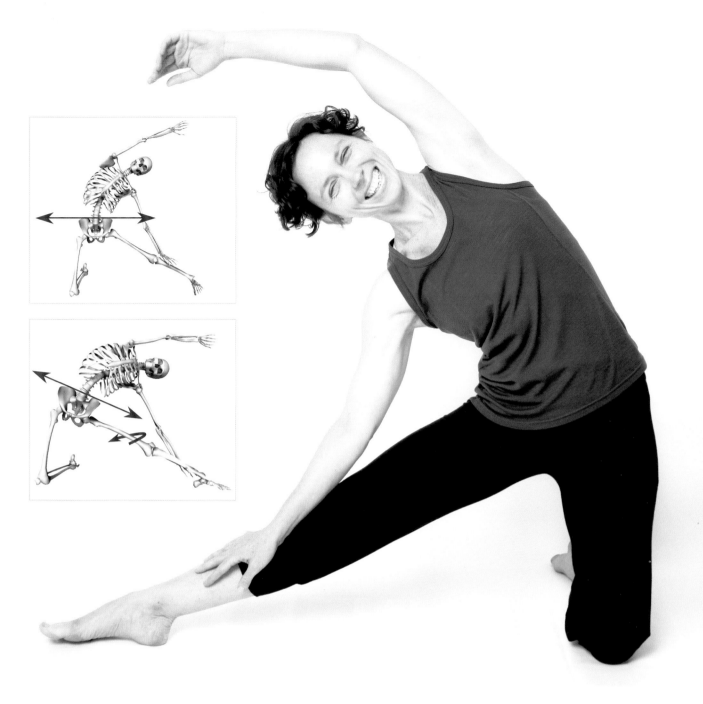

Kneeling side bend
Parigasana or gate pose

The kneeling side bend, or *Parigasana,* is another useful side bend, although once again gravity tends to be the prime mover, which means that the side-bending pattern is less likely to be employed. However, it is helpful to ensure that movement takes place in the spine rather than in the hip joints. With the hips stable, it is unlikely that shearing forces will develop above the sacrum.

This is true though only when the foot of the extended leg points forwards. In this position the greater trochanter of the femur prevents side-bending of the pelvis, ensuring motion takes place in the spine. However, when the extended leg is externally rotated, the greater

trochanter moves backwards and allows the pelvis to tip sideways, as it does in standing. When this happens, there is a deep stretch to the adductors of the extended leg, but the risk of side-shearing at the lumbosacral and sacroiliac joints increases. For an experienced practitioner, who is well accustomed to examining patterns of movement, this presents less of a problem.

Having the feet forward in the wide-stride standing position does not prevent side-tipping of the pelvis in the same way as it does in the kneeling side bend. In the kneeling side bend, the extended leg is abducted much further than in wide-stride standing, which brings the greater trochanter much closer to the ilium.

EXTENSION POSTURES
Getting upright

These are the later developmental movements of the child, and the movements that enable quadruped mammal to run fast and climb over difficult terrain.

In the human being, extension movements happen most easily in the lumbar and cervical spine. We should remember that both the lumbar and the cervical curve are acquired – we aren't born with them; rather, they are created as the baby starts to employ the tonic extensor reflex patterns, and later as they progress on to two legs.

Although genetics will go some way to determining how deep the lumbar and cervical curves are, how we deal with extension movements will be equally if not more important.

The thoracic spine, because of its attached rib cage and the elongated spinal processes, has much more difficulty moving into extension; its natural tendency is towards flexion, and in the population at large this drift towards flexion of the upper back is almost ubiquitous. It is, therefore, important to realise that the main issue with back bends is not how far we can bend backwards but how we bring the upper spine from flexion to uprightness.

Human beings spend very little of their lives in extension, and when they do it requires much more effort than flexion. For this reason, it is unwise to sustain them.

Back bends, then, are less about trying to bend back as far as possible, and more to do with teaching the body how to distribute the pattern as evenly as possible. It is important to recognise that people who have a great deal of

BELOW
The back bend performed by this contortionist is done completely from the lumbar spine. This hyper flexibility is a genetic trait and no amount of practice will enable an average person to do it

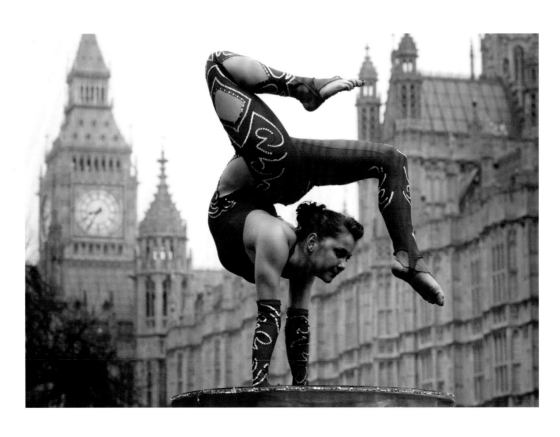

extension in the lower back are born like that. It is something determined by the thickness of the intervertebral discs.

Acrobats and contortionists have very thick discs which allow a great deal of movement, particularly in the lumbar spine. No amount of practice will turn someone with genetically thinner discs into someone with thicker ones, so trying to emulate the deeper back bends if your body is not built that way will only end in tears.

There are two places in the body that really don't like to extend: the hip joint and the thoracic spine. As these areas stiffen, more and more is asked of the lumbar spine and cervical spine when we need to lean back, causing more compression at these already vulnerable areas.

If the man illustrated on the right is a cloud spotter, he's going to need regular visits to his osteopath.

As we have discussed, the limitations in movement of the thoracic spine are largely due to the attachment of the ribs and the limitation of the spinous processes.

At the hip joint, extension is resisted by two main structures. These are the iliopsoas muscle and the iliofemoral ligaments.

Both these structures are slackened off when we are in the all-fours position and tighten as we stand up. Again, it is interesting to reflect on the evolutionary and an individual's' progress from all fours to the upright position. See drawing on page 80.

In moving to the bipedal position (from a quadrupedal one) the area that needs to change the most is the hip joint; failure to open at the hip will put greater demands on the lumbar spine.

The hip ligaments create stability at the hip joint. They are short, tough ligaments that bind the femur to the pelvis. They look like one strong

Human beings spend very little of their lives in extension, and when they do it requires much more effort than flexion

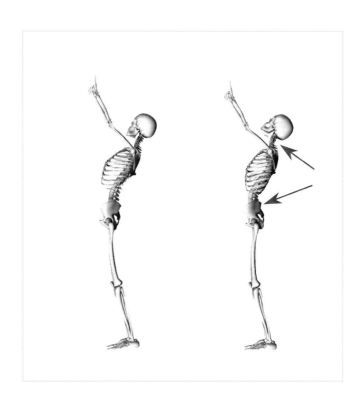

ABOVE
If the person (skeleton) on the right were cloud spotting, he would certainly develop neck and low back pain

band of connective tissue, but can be separated into three main groups: the ischiofemoral ligament; the pubofemoral ligament and the iliofemoral ligament – attaching the femur to the ischium, pubic bone and ilium respectively. In standing, the iliofemoral ligament provides the resistance to further extension and prevents the pelvis from tipping backwards.

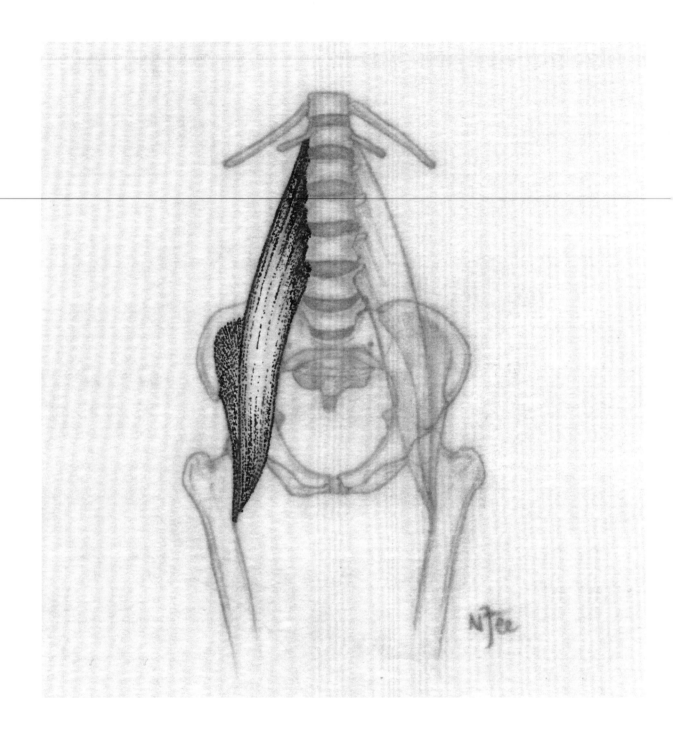

The iliopsoas muscle

Much has been written about the iliopsoas because of its crucial role in maintaining pelvic balance. It is really two muscles with a common insertion into the lesser trochanter of the femur.

The iliacus originates from the inner surface of the ilium, while the psoas has a broad origin from the first to the fifth lumbar. Together these are the most powerful flexors of the hip joint.

It is debatable whether the iliofemoral ligament or the iliopsoas muscle provide the most significant resistance to extension, and my guess is that it varies from individual to individual. What might make a difference, and what is significant about this muscle, is its role in the startle reflex. When we are scared we tend to contract certain muscles to protect ourselves – the same muscles that we have used for hundreds of thousands of years.

We protect our vulnerable neck with the powerful neck extensors and scapula elevators, and the soft belly with the hip flexors. This is a deeply embedded response, and when we are anxious these muscles will have tightened before we know it. This unconscious tightening

ABOVE
The iliopsoas inhabits a central position in the body, stabilising the pelvis and modifying the lumbar curve

is responsible for much of the neck, shoulder, and lower back pain that keep body-workers so busy these days.

Chronic use of this iliopsoas muscle will, inevitably, tighten and shorten it. So, paying attention to this area is vital if we are going to free the lumbar spine, especially in back bends.

If we exaggerate slightly the effect of tension in the iliopsoas we can see more clearly its effect on the lumbar spine. The position illustrated by the top skeleton (right) with the tight hip flexors is likely to suffer more compressive effects in the lower back than the position illustrated by the skeleton illustrated below. And of course, if back bends are initiated from the position on the left, one is simply asking for trouble.

How we deal with this is not as straightforward as merely stretching; we must first learn how to break an unhelpful pattern of use.

Extension movements

Extension movements, then, are intended to integrate thoracic movement into the movements of the lumbar and cervical spine. To do this, the thoracic erector spinae need to be strong and active when required and be able to relax and release when not required. The same must apply to the antagonists, particularly pectoralis major and minor. In the lumbar region we have seen that the deep hip flexors need to develop freedom to release, namely the iliopsoas and the deep hip ligaments.

Another important consideration when attempting back-bending movements is the effect of the breath on the spine, particularly the thoracic spine, to which the ribs (which we need for breathing) are attached.

The rib cage is the major limiting factor in all movements of the thoracic spine, and it is a useful exercise to see how they influence the spine as we breathe.

When we breathe in, the ribs elevate. The lower ribs tend to widen in a bucket handle fashion and we feel ourselves widen in the lower trunk. The upper ribs and breast bone lift forwards and upwards in pump-handle fashion, and we feel ourselves get deeper from front to back in the upper part of the trunk.

Movement of the spine is often missed in this action. When we breathe in, the ribs do indeed lift and push the breast bone forwards, but the thoracic spine is at the same time pushed backwards. Every inhalation is accompanied by a gentle forward bending of the thoracic spine, while on every exhalation the opposite happens, and the spine moves towards extension. There is no exception to this action, so it makes absolute sense to move into extension postures as we breathe out, if our intention is to access the thoracic spine.

Anything else will be going against the intelligence of the body; if we move into back bends on the in breath, while the thoracic spine is flexing, we will simply push the back bend into our lumbars – the very thing we are hoping to avoid.

RIGHT
The effect that tension in the iliopsoas has on the lumbar curve can be seen in the image of the upper skeleton

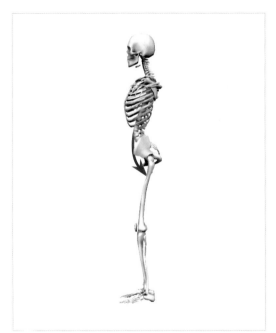

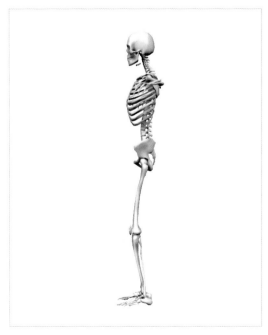

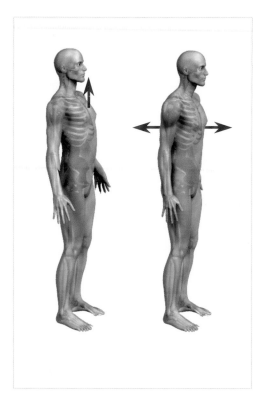

Neither lifting the ribs (left) nor simply breathing in (right) facilitate extension in the thoracic spine

Breathing in v. lifting the ribs

As we breathe in, the ribs elevate, deepening the chest from front to back. The breastbone moves forward and the spine moves backwards. There may also be a slight deepening of the lumbar curve, by virtue of the pull of the diaphragm on the front of the lumbar spine as it contracts.

When we lift the ribs, something we can do without breathing, we do so by pulling up with the muscles that attach the rib cage to the skull and neck – the scalenes and the sternocleidomastoid. This is accompanied by a pulling down of the lower back via the quadratus lumborum and the lower erector spinae, probably the iliocostalis lumborum.

Neither the inhalation nor the action of lifting the ribs support extension movements of the thoracic spine, because the lumbar curve deepens in both these actions and we want to avoid over bending from here. Of course the reverse happens when we exhale, and the curves of the spine tend to straighten out.

As has been discussed there is a tendency towards stiffness in the thoracic spine, and often – but not always – this is accompanied by a movement towards flexion; the "dowager's hump" is an example of this.

When the upper thoracic spine becomes stiff it is often difficult to reintroduce movement into this area. One way of doing this is through the use of the head and neck.

To understand this more clearly a diversion into anatomy may be useful. When we are on all fours there are a number of muscles that can support the head and neck, but just two major ones limit their work to the head and neck. These muscles are called splenius capitus, and splenius cervices. They run from the base of the skull, and the middle of the neck respectively, and both insert into the mid thoracic region. In quadrupeds these muscles are very large and have to support the head and neck all the time, in humans their job is less arduous. However, understanding their role in quadrupeds can be very helpful, especially when we are on all fours. When we are in this position it is useful to imagine your neck being supported from the middle of your shoulders. When you do this you remind yourself of the muscles that can easily "fall asleep".

In back bends, when you lift from this area, the thoracic spine "wakes up" and you start to move a part of the spine that can easily seize up. In fact it is useful to imagine most prone back bends being initiated from the head and neck ie from between the shoulder blades, and the rest of the spine being invited to join in.

BELOW Splenius capitus runs from the base of the skull to between the shoulder blades, and splenius cervices run from the middle of the neck to the mid thoracic

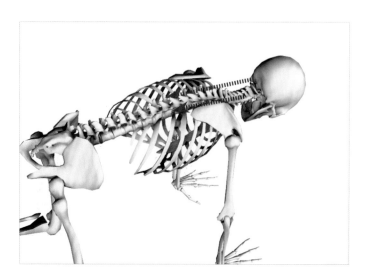

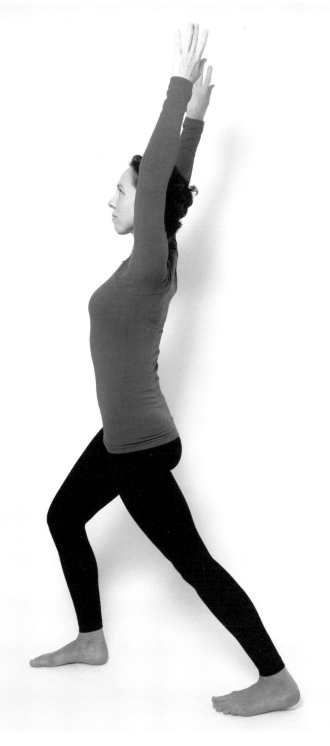

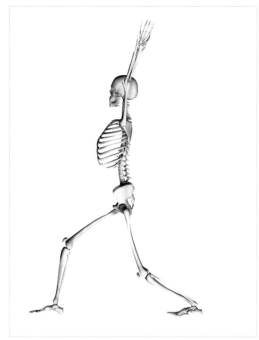

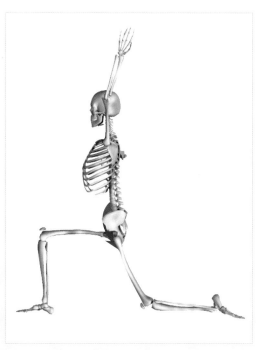

Standing back bend
Virabhadrasana One or first warrior pose

Of all the standing poses, the only true back bend is the first warrior pose, also known as *Virabhadrasana One*.

Extension at the hip is felt clearly in the kneeling version of this posture, where the lumbar spine is protected as the hip extends.

Bending from the lower back is not the main point here; rather the intention should be to extend the hip, and then for the upper spine to become more involved in extension. This is best achieved, as in most extension movements, by leading with the eyes and head. It is also important that the pelvis is facing forwards, so that the lumbar spine extends from the pelvis without rotation or side-bending.

When this pose is brought into the standing position, a complication occurs; the knee joints can now bend, so that the psoas will no longer be lengthening. Consequently, the point of the pose can be lost.

The feet need to stay parallel, to prevent rotational forces in the knee. When this pose is stable and balanced, exhalation provides the impetus to develop the back bend into the thoracic spine, creating an even curve from the hip joint to the base of the skull.

ABOVE
When kneeling, lengthening the hip flexors is straightforward (lower inset) however, when we stand, if the knee bends, the length is taken away from the hip flexors making the posture less effective (top inset)

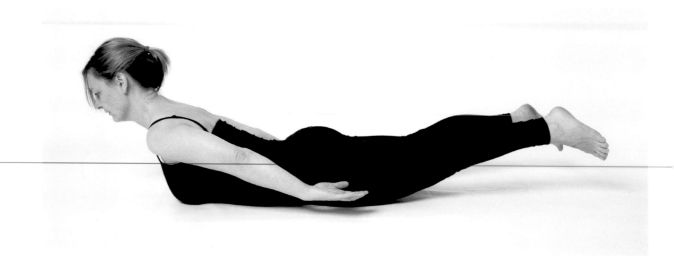

Prone back bend
Salabhasana

This is the most fundamental of back bends. It engages the extensor muscles in a patterned way, so that all the muscles of spinal extension are engaged, and the antagonists are relaxed.

The muscles used here are the hamstrings and gluteals to extend the legs, the erector spinae to extend the spine, and the lower trapezius to anchor the scapular down.

As with any patterned activity we are interested in the way the movement is distributed throughout the body. Again we need to remember that the difficult places to move from are the hip joint and the thoracic spine. We can all extend from the neck and lower back, so pursuing those movements too far is pointless. At the hip, we need to differentiate between the hip joint and the lumbar spine. If we can't find the movement from the hip, we will almost certainly bend more from the lumbars.

When movement comes from the hip joint, the lumbar spine is protected. This can only happen if there is enough length and release in both the iliofemoral ligament and the iliopsoas muscle.

However, when movement is restricted at the hip joint it will be the lumbar spine that has to bend, in so doing compressing an area that is often over-compressed anyway to (below left). In attempting to lift against the resistance of the hip flexors, we frequently find ourselves bending from another "easy place", namely the neck.

When practised with attention to the distribution of movement, this posture helps develop an even tone in the extensor muscles of the body, while at the same time encouraging a release of the flexor muscles. It is the only back bend to act in this way, and it is, therefore, an important posture for restoring and maintaining a good balance between flexion and extension. It is not how far you bend that's important, but how well-distributed your pattern of movement is.

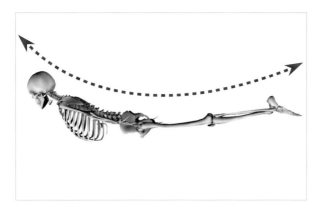

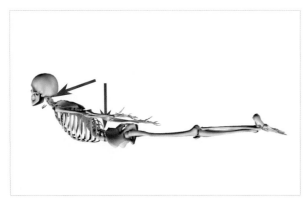

Hands-to-ankle prone back bend

Dhanurasana or the bow

At first glance, this posture does not look too dissimilar to the prone back bend. It is however quite different.

The muscles engaged in the bow are mainly the quadriceps, gluteals and hamstrings. The intention of this posture is to passively bend the upper back using the muscles of the legs.

The gluteals (predominately) and hamstrings (slightly) lift the legs, as they do in the prone back bend, but the chest is lifted, and the thoracic spine extended by the pulling of the feet away from the head, via the action of the quadriceps.

A difficult pose to perform well, it allows the back to be extended without the potentially compressive effects of tightening the erector spinae. This is a particularly difficult job for the rectus femoris, the only bi-articular quadricep, as it has to both contract to extend the knee, and lengthen over the hip joint as the hip is extended.

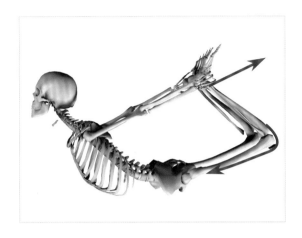

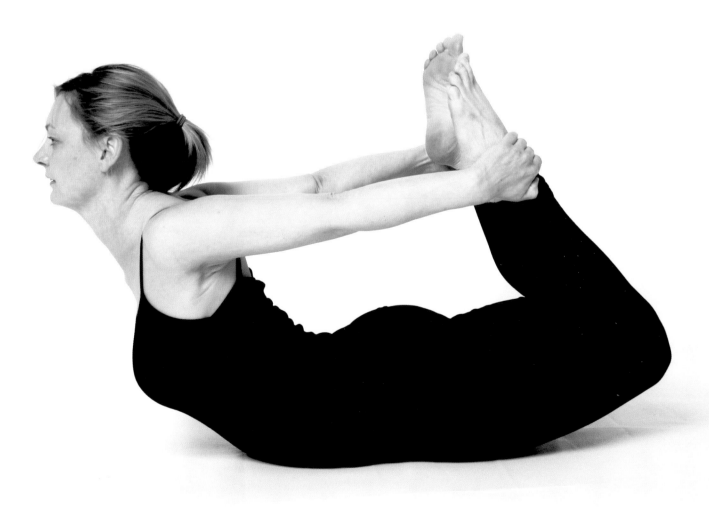

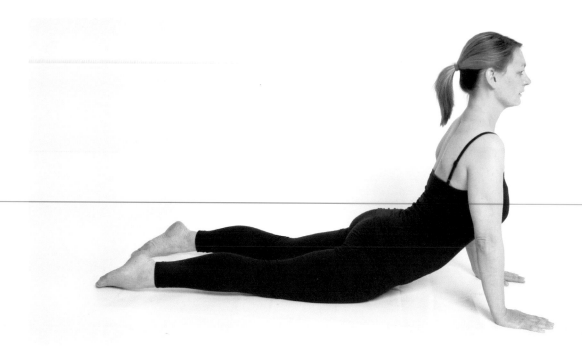

The cobra
Bhujangasana

This posture is another prone back bend, but this time the arms are used to take the lumbar spine into extension.

As with all back bends, the key areas are the hip joint and the thoracic spine. It is all too easy in this pose to lever yourself into the lumbar spine and cause considerable compression. The full posture, where the arms are straight under the shoulders, demands a lot of freedom in the lower spine and hip. Unless you have this, the cobra can cause problems in the lower back.

If compression in the lumbar spine makes this pose uncomfortable a solution is to support yourself on the elbows in what is sometimes known as sphinx pose. This reduces the amount of bend in the lumbar spine, but still makes available the bend in the thoracic spine.

Whether you practise cobra or the modified

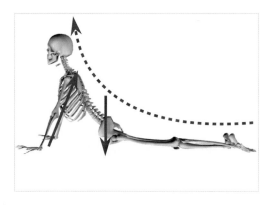

sphinx pose it is important to note that the work of the shoulder girdle is to provide support, ensuring the shoulders are drawn down away from the ears, rather than forcing the thoracic spine into extension.. Forcing the chest forwards by pulling the shoulders back only creates tension in an area that we are trying to free.

This posture is often taught on the inhalation, largely I think, because of the feeling of expansion it brings at the front of the chest. However, as we have seen, the thoracic spine itself is moving into flexion during inhalation; if you move into this posture while you breathe in, you will force the back bend to come from the lumbars, which we want to avoid.

If going up on the exhalation feels confusing initially, try turning your attention to the spine between the shoulder blades, and really feeling how the spine moves as you breathe. It quite soon becomes apparent that the exhalation, and not the in breath, facilitates the bend.

Perhaps a more satisfactory way of approaching cobra is to lower yourself from the plank pose. When coming into it from this direction it is important that the pelvis is free and not held in some habit. This approach allows you to lower to a point that the lower spine can tolerate, and there is less chance of levering yourself uncomfortably into the lumbar spine.

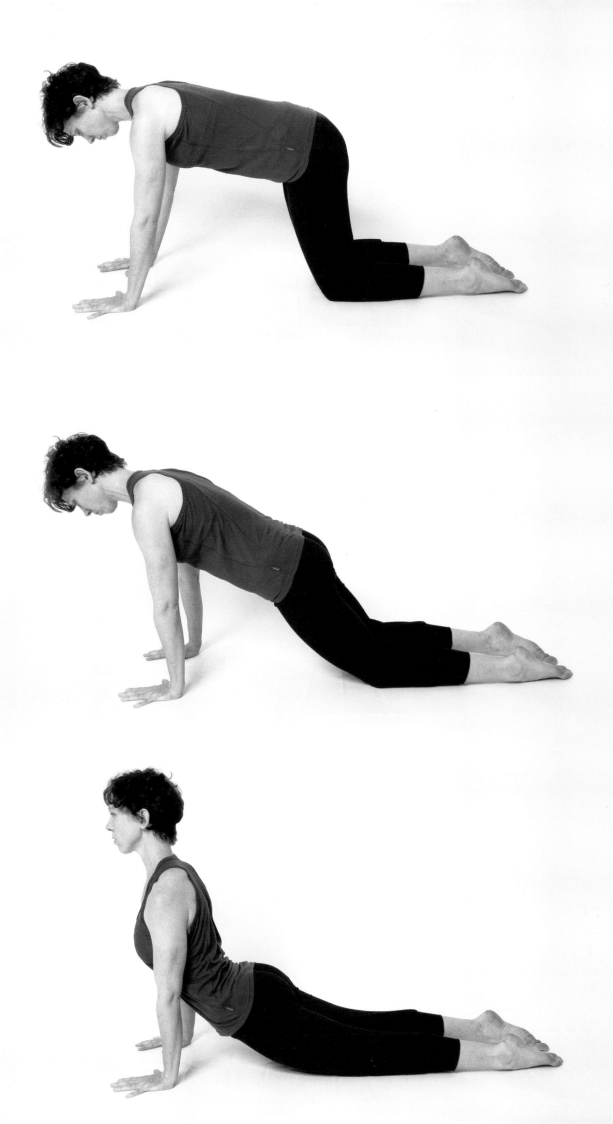

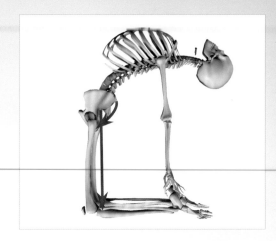

Kneeling back bend
Ustrasana or the camel

This postures requires a great deal of attention to prevent compression in the lumbar and cervical spine. The lumbar spine is more vulnerable to compression in the kneeling back bend because the quadriceps are stretched over the knee joint and therefore exert more of a downward pull on their origin at the front of the pelvis.

Also, because the knee is bent, the hamstrings are slackened and lose much of the power needed to tether the pelvis from below; and so the gluteals will probably have to work a bit harder. As with all back bends, the intention is to involve the thoracic spine, and again movement on the exhalation is essential if an integrated movement is to be achieved.

To my mind this is an advanced posture but, it is useful because when the head is able to drop back it can encourage the upper thoracic spine to participate in extension. However, the hip, lower back and mid thoracic spine need to have a certain level of extension before this movement becomes beneficial. If you try and drop the head back before the rest of the spine can accommodate the movement you risk compressing the delicate blood vessels at the base of the skull. If on the other hand you keep the head looking forward you take the upper thoracic spine into flexion – the opposite of what is required, making the posture rather pointless.

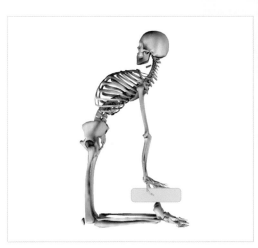

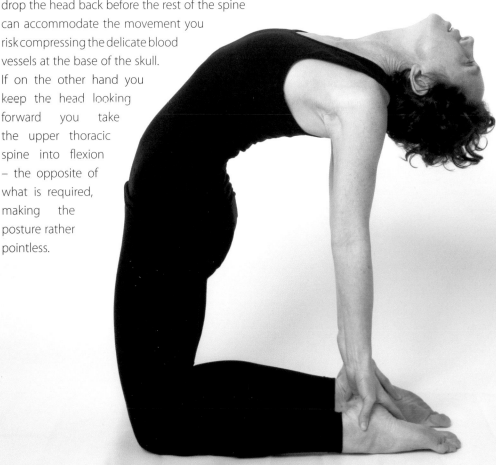

TOP
The gluteals and hamstrings provide the anchoring for the pelvis from below

Extension postures – getting upright

Kneeling supine back bend
Paryankasana or fish pose variation

BELOW
Ideally, the weight of the head can be used to help the upper back move into extension (centre). It is a mistake to pull the head back causing compression at the base of the skull (bottom)

This is one of the more difficult poses in to do well, and is certainly not a beginner's pose. Good understanding is required to perform it well, because done carelessly it risks considerable compression at a vulnerable area at the base of the skull.

Yet the kneeling supine back bend is worth working towards, because it challenges an area of the upper thoracic spine that few poses reach. It can be practised with the legs in the hero pose (*Virasana*), in the lotus position (*Padmasana*) or with the legs out straight.

The intention of this pose is to take the upper thoracic spine into extension using the weight of the head to help bring the upper spine with it. What you must avoid is pulling in and actively shortening the back of the neck. When performed well the entire spine is involved in this back bend, not just the neck and lumbars.

One of the major points of this pose is to allow the head to drop downward. This helps the very stiff area around the seventh cervical, and the first and second thoracic vertebra to move a little into extension. Getting this area to participate in extension goes a long way to relieving neck pain.

If the upper spine cannot participate in the back bend the neck will have to do more, and serious compression can then take place at the base of the skull. This can create a similar problem to that described in the kneeling back bend, with the delicate vertebral arteries risking compression.

The kneeling supine back bend can be a very useful pose to free the stiffest part of the spine, but this can only happen if there is reasonable flexibility in the rest of the thoracic spine. It is a potentially dangerous pose if attempted when the upper thoracic spine is in flexion or cannot readily move into extension.

The kneeling back bend and the kneeling supine back bend are part of the same family of back bends as they have the potential to allow the head and neck to mobilise the stiff upper thoracic areas. As we have seen, it is very useful to get this part of the spine moving so the extension movement does not become fragmented.

This distinguishes them from the first back bends we looked at, those performed from the prone position, which require the spinal extensor muscles to pull us up against gravity. These are the only true patterned back bends, where the extensor muscles of the spine are asked to perform the job of extension.

Cobra and the wheel pose, which we will look at next, work in a different way again. These postures use the arms to move the lumbar spine into extension so here we are looking at the distribution of the extension curve, rather than working on patterned movement.

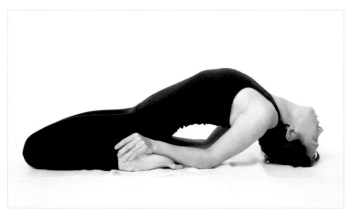

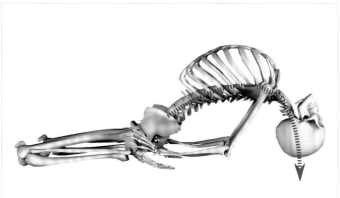

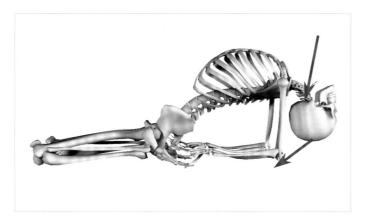

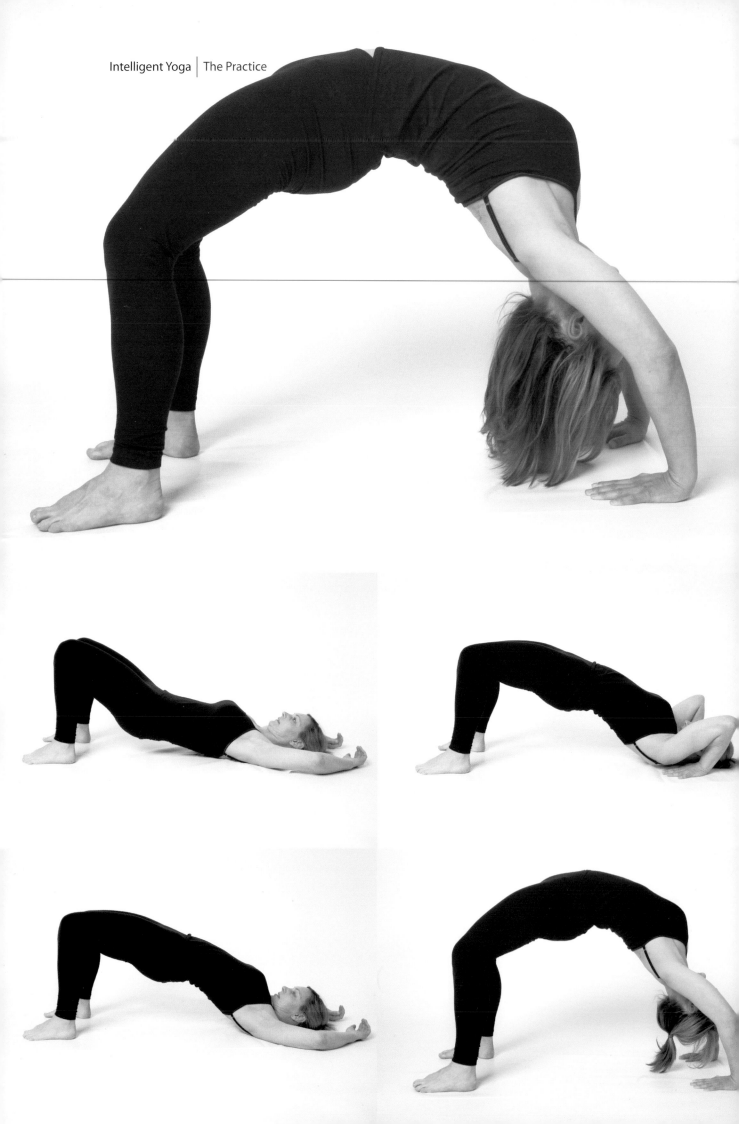

The wheel

Urdhva Dhanurasana

This is potentially one of the most beautiful yoga postures. In some ways it shouldn't really be in the back bend section; when done from the floor it is more about the transmission of force through the skeleton, and not at all about trying to back bend. The movement is delivered into the spine by pushing into the floor with the hands and feet. It is the ability to release the hips, spine and shoulders while you push into the floor that creates the back bend shape.

As with the previous back bends, sufficient length in the iliopsoas is essential. The upper spine needs to be mobile, and freedom in the shoulders is important (you need enough length in the latissimus dorsi). Our areas of freedom vary, which will influence the way our version of the posture looks.

Preparation for this asana is important and its initiation can appear paradoxical; to lift the pelvis we have to push down through the feet, making the start of this pose feel more like a forward bend.

Before you start, it is worth spending some time settling the body quietly into the floor and noticing what happens when you start to push your feet into the floor. If we don't interfere, the first thing that will happen is that the pelvis rolls under and the belly deepens. This is because when we push with our feet we engage the extensor muscles of the hip. This, through agonist/antagonist pairing, relaxes the hip flexors, which is an ideal start for any back bend.

The belly will deepen if we have managed to relax the muscles around the ribs and upper spine, and with the ribs slightly wider, the diaphragm draws up a little, and the belly follows. We find a gentle but natural Uddiyana Bandha appearing spontaneously, without intention.

As the feet press down, the belly drops and the pelvis rolls under. The spine can lift off the ground vertebra by vertebra.

As the pose develops, the hips are lifted higher by the action of the hip and knee extensors. The rest of the body needs to remain relaxed to reduce resistance to the back bend. It is a mistake at this point to lift the ribs and engage the spinal extensors because the groin then has to close, and the movement will tend to come from the lower back.

For many people it is not worth bringing the hands into the push-down position until the hips are fully open. The higher the hips are, the less work the arms will need to do. Many people believe they are not strong enough to lift up into this posture, but usually it is simply that they are unable to lift the hips sufficiently to get any purchase with the arms.

When you finally move into this position, by pushing down into the floor with the feet and hands, the back bend is distributed through the hips, spine and shoulders.

it is the ability to release the hips, spine and shoulders while you push into the floor that creates the back bend shape

If the iliopsoas is tight, but the shoulders and upper spine are free, the pose will shift to the easy areas over the hands

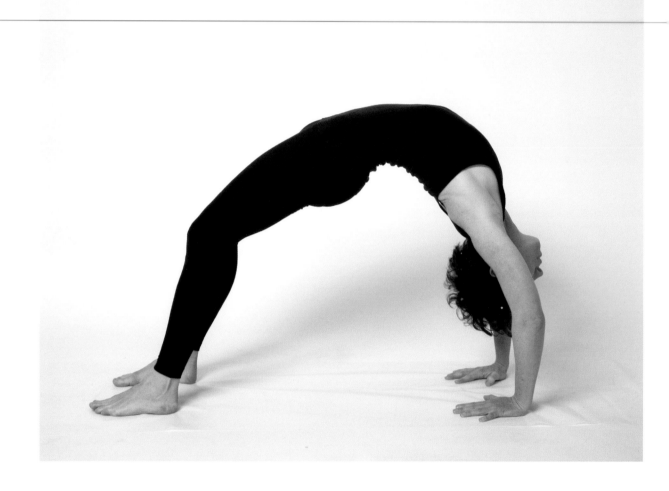

If the iliopsoas is tight, but the shoulders and upper spine are free, the pose will shift to the easy areas over the hands. It is not useful to keep going in this direction, as the hips will stay tight while the shoulders get over stretched.

If, on the other hand, the shoulders are held back by tightness in the latissimus dorsi, but the hips are free, the pose will shift the other way over towards the feet. This person will need to learn to move more over the hands if she is going to balance the distribution of extension through the body.

If both the hips and shoulders are tight, it will be difficult to lift off the ground. It is usually only strong men who push through this resistance, unfortunately at the expense of their lower back, which has to try to make up the difference.

In many postures where we are lifting up, we forget that the only way to do this is by paying attention to how we go down. In the wheel pose we can only lift the body by pressing down through the feet and hands.

If we are interested in improving the quality of our posture work, then paying close attention to the way we meet the floor is essential. In all aspects of posture work, when something lifts, it is always preceded by something else going down. If you want a part of the body to lift, try to recognise what has to drop first in order to facilitate the lift. This way you are more likely to put effort into the right areas and avoid straining.

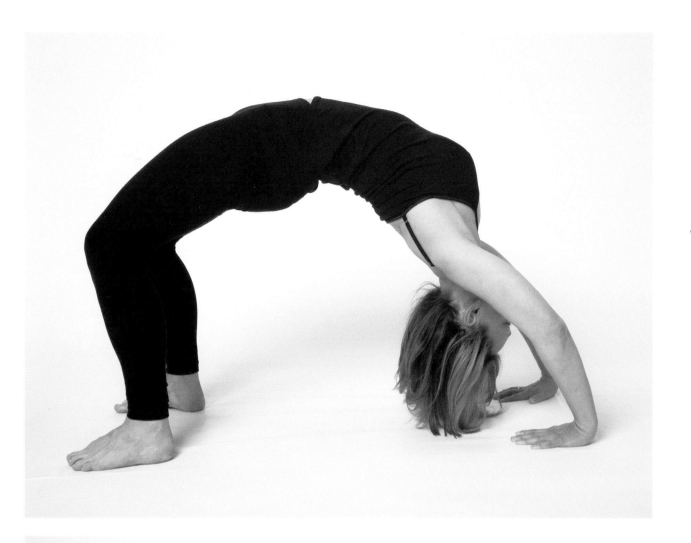

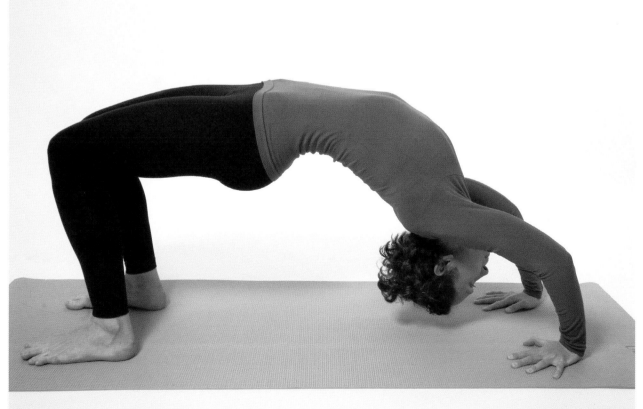

FI FXION

A consequence of being upright

The muscles of flexion and extension must balance each other if standing, sitting or moving are to be comfortable. Somewhere between three and four million years ago our ancestors moved out of the trees and onto the savannah. Standing erect brought many advantages, but it also meant we had to do a lot of bending. We had to lift things from the floor into the upright position and carry them. The constant process of bending and lifting honed the efficiency of this movement, and on the back of the body we have a great deal of connective tissue that supports the weight of the body as we bend forward. The nature of the hamstrings is revealed in their names: semimembranosus and semitendinosus tells you that much of these muscles are made of tendon and fascia, and are well equipped to deal with the tensile forces they receive when we bend forwards. The lower back is enveloped in a broad sheet of fascia called the lumbodorsal

fascia that runs down and broadens over the gluteal muscles, again evolved to support the weight of the trunk in flexion.

Yoga involves many forward bends. Most flexion movements are gravity assisted and therefore tend to use the eccentrically contracting extensor muscles to control the movement. However, the connective tissue previously described takes much of the effort from these muscles when full flexion of the spine is reached..

Muscles of Flexion

Not all flexion movement is assisted by gravity, as it is in the case of bending towards the ground. If we are moving into flexion against gravity then the flexor muscles are called into play; namely the iliopsoas, the main hip flexors, and the abdominal muscles, which are the main flexors of the trunk.

We must be clear here that the deepest

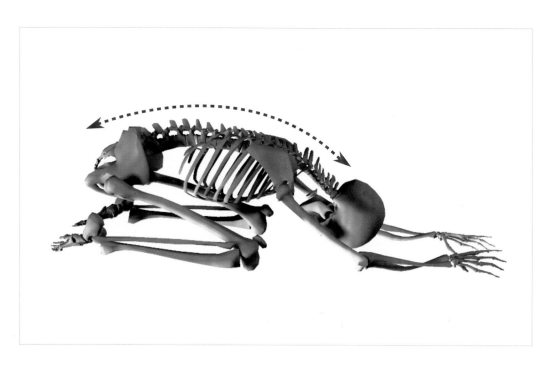

LEFT
An even lengthening of the spinal muscles is desirable in child's pose.

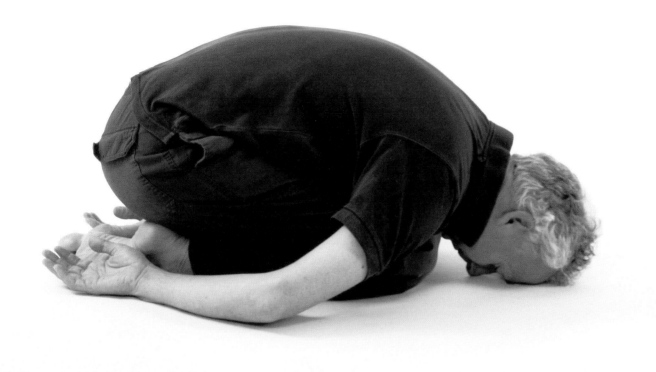

abdominal muscle group, the transverse abdominals, are not flexors; rather, they are supporting muscles for the abdominal and pelvic contents, and by virtue of this they also support the lumbar spine in the upright position.

Every time we lift a leg, we engage the iliopsoas. It is a muscle that is rarely under-used. Its tendency if anything is overuse, thanks to its participation in the startle reflex. The iliopsoas also has a tendency to shortness, in those of us who spend a lot of time sitting.

The abdominals are a different kettle of fish being, as they are, muscles we rarely have cause to use these days. The abdominals help us to sit up from a lying position, and would once have been used to help swing our bodies upwards when climbing. With few of us engaging in such activity, there is a marked tendency for

abdominal muscles to weaken, especially in women who have had children and whose muscles have been subjected to continued stretch.

We also have flexor muscles in the neck, but these are comparatively weak as the head will want to fall forwards rather than backwards in the upright position. This is because the fulcrum of the head on the neck is behind the head's centre of gravity. Thanks to this fact the main muscles supporting the neck are the extensors. Nevertheless, understanding the neck flexors is useful. Babies develop tone in the abdominals when lying on their back and lifting their bodies into a mini sit up. This is a good starting point from which to explore the muscles of flexion: lying on the back and finding out how we can lift the ends of the body.

Half boat pose

Ardha Navasana

This posture clarifies the patterned response, the entire body coming into flexion using the flexor muscles. It is the counterpoint to the prone back bend; achieving both poses with equal ease, suggests a balance in these muscles groups.

The abdominal muscles bring the ribs closer to the pelvis, and in so doing flex the lumbar spine. The rectus abdominus is the most important of the group, but the internal and external obliques will also be busy.

The abdominals cannot lift the legs; rather, this is primarily the work of the iliopsoas, with the rectus femoris playing a secondary role in the movement. The three vasti lift the lower leg by straightening the knee.

The head and neck demand closer attention, as lifting the weight of the head is often an arduous task. The muscles involved are delicate and their task is complex. We will look more closely at these later

Flexion – a consequence of being upright

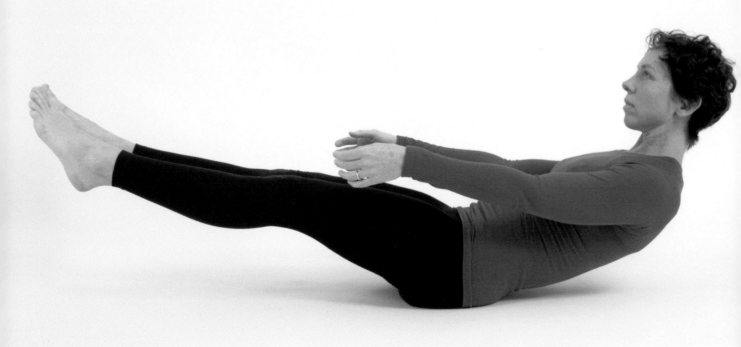

Supine flexion or V-sitting

Paripuna Navasana

Although this pose is similar to the previous one there are some crucial differences. In supine flexion the legs are lifted higher and the lower back is encouraged to straighten, moving it from the more flexed position of half boat pose to a straight one. Drawing the spine in and lifting the legs are both actions of the iliopsoas, so this muscle has to work very hard in this pose. The abdominals also have to work to keep the front of the rib cage and pelvis from moving away from each other. Because this pose requires such activity in the iliopsoas I have some reservations about teaching it as many people overuse this muscle anyway, perhaps the most import thing in relation to the above postures is that eventually they feel equally easy, one not dominating the other. One other point with this pose, is that people with tight hamstrings will find it even trickier, as they will have to overcome the tension in these muscles on top of everything else.

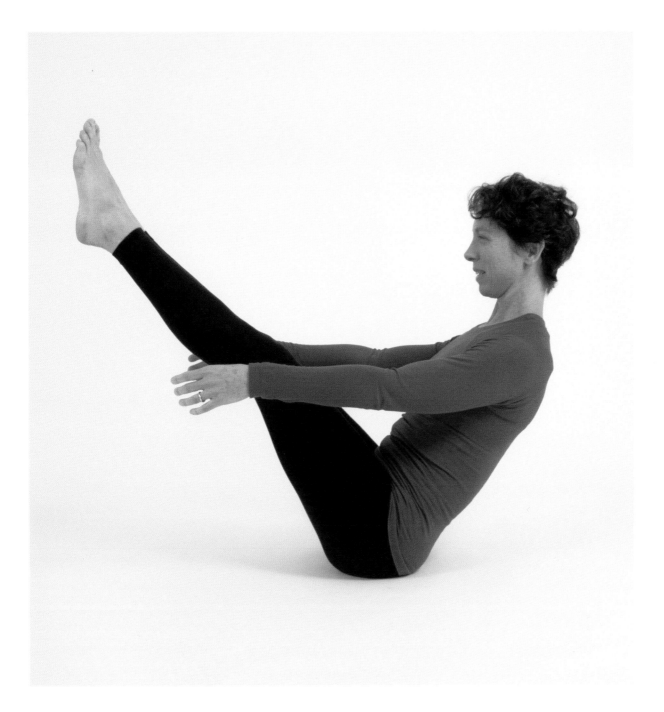

Flexion – a consequence of being upright

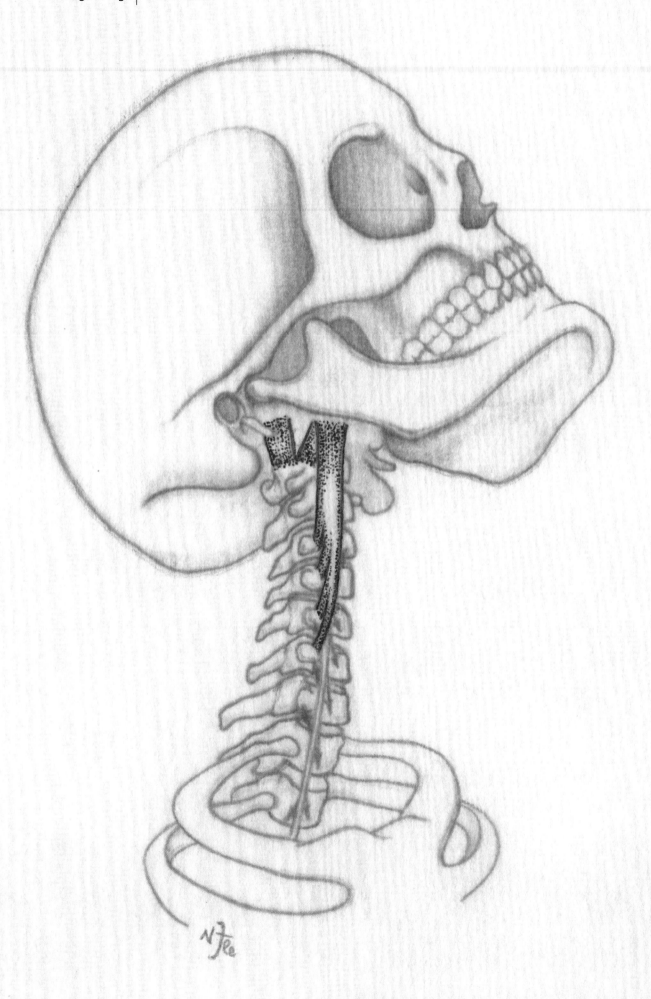

The deep flexor muscles of the neck

These are an interesting and, to my mind, important group of muscles to familiarise yourself with. Although these muscles are small their function is significant.

Ideally, looking down should start deep in the neck. In the upright position, the deep flexor muscles of the neck have very little to do as gravity does most of the work. Nevertheless, an awareness of their action is helpful. Their job is to draw the front of the head down and reduce the lordotic curve in the neck. When these deep muscles are consciously thought about, the large antagonist extensor muscles tend to quiet down.

I sometimes imagine that these small flexor muscles whisper important things to our nervous system, while the large extensors are shouting loudly, grabbing too much attention with their alarmist talk.

If we just stand for a while and listen attentively to the voice of the deep neck flexors, and their gentle request for the front of the neck to draw in towards the back of the neck, the blustering neck extensors, because of their antagonistic role, become slowly subdued.

It is lovely to feel the sense of release of the skull from the neck, and to develop a "nodding dog" feeling. This sense of depth within the neck is very useful in standing, and becomes even more important in the flexion movements.

If we don't have a sense of this, it is all too easy to involve the larger external muscles, the ones that can cause so much misery with the aches of overuse.

Of the deep neck flexors, there is a particularly interesting little group of muscles running up the front of the spine and attaching to the occiput – just in front of the foramen magnum (the hole in the base of the skull that accepts the central nervous system). These very deep muscles on the front of the cervical spine tend to gently straighten the neck and flex the head slightly. As they act, the antagonists at the back of the skull, the rectus capitus posterior, and the associated sub-occipital muscles, will relax.

Small as it is, the rectus capitus posterior is highly significant, given its connective tissue attachment to the dura mater, the membrane surrounding the spinal cord and brain.

Continued tension in this small muscle is transmitted directly to the tissues surrounding our central nervous system. It is difficult to know what the effect of inappropriate tension here would be but it could be profound, with headaches an obvious possibility. In yoga, particularly in the standing postures, just how we balance the head on the neck is very important.

Imagining the rectus capitus anterior doing its job correctly brings our attention to deep within the neck, a place we don't usually think about. It diverts attention from the large outer muscles, so we don't risk pulling the chin down with the larger external muscles, which will simply pull our head down more on to our neck.

In all flexion movements of the head on the neck we need to try to think of the movement starting deep in the neck, maintaining space in those tight little areas at the base of the skull.

LEFT
Rectus capitus anterior and longus colli

(Illustration adapted from a drawing in IA Kapandji's book *The Physiology of the Joints*, Churchill Livingston, 1974)

BELOW
Rectus capitus posterior (red) and its connection to the dura mater (blue)

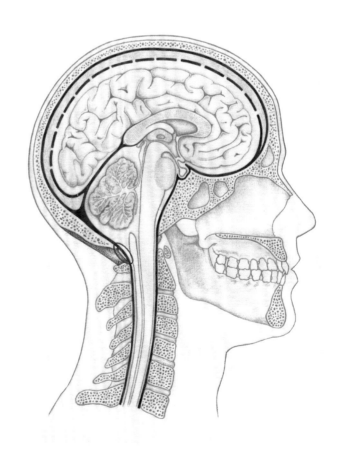

Flexion – a consequence of being upright

Spinal rolling

The initiation of this pose requires work in the hip flexors, namely the iliopsoas (top right), to bring the legs off the floor. If the hamstrings are long enough, the quadriceps are then used at this point to straighten the knee. This is useful as it helps to shift the centre of gravity across the shoulders as you roll up.

To bring the pelvis off the floor and to start to curl the spine upwards requires the use of the abdominal muscles, as well as flexibility and release in the lumbar spine (middle right). When the thighs pass the centre of gravity, the iliopsoas is no longer required as the force of gravity now brings the legs over the head.

When commencing spinal rolling it is the abdominal muscles that lift you off the floor. They have also to lift the weight of the legs. The abdominals have to continue to work until the centre of gravity has passed the shoulders; this will be easier if it is possible to straighten the legs.

Once the abdominal muscles have lifted the pelvis off the floor, the iliopsoas is no longer required to flex the hip, as gravity now does this. If the abdominal muscles are weak, the muscles of arm extension are substituted when they rest beside the trunk; initially the latissimus dorsi, but then, and dominantly, the posterior deltoid.

When the body goes past the centre of gravity, the abdominals are no longer engaged, and the extensor muscles of the back are now active (bottom right).

Rolling through the spine brings flexibility to the back and encourages the muscles of flexion to act while the extensor muscles lengthen. Once the gravity line has been passed, the abdominals relax and the back extensors (mainly the erector spinae) take over the job of resisting gravity.

If it is difficult to achieve this movement with the abdominals, you can push down with the arms to help. However, it is still important to try and curl the spine, so that the nervous system learns something of the process.

In flexion the three main rules are that firstly, the chin stays in towards the body thanks to the action of the deep neck flexors (or gravity); secondly, the low front ribs stay in, thanks to the abdominals; and thirdly, the pelvis tucks under, again thanks to the abdominals - the main spinal muscles of flexion.

When we turn ourselves over so we are prone, with our faces facing down as in child's pose, gravity becomes the prime mover in flexion. In this position, the flexor muscles are usually quiet.

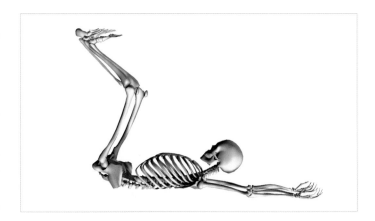

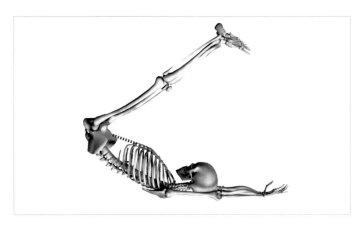

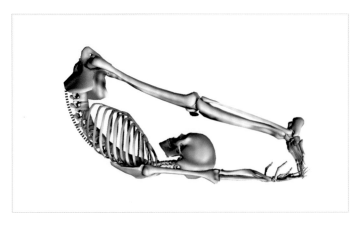

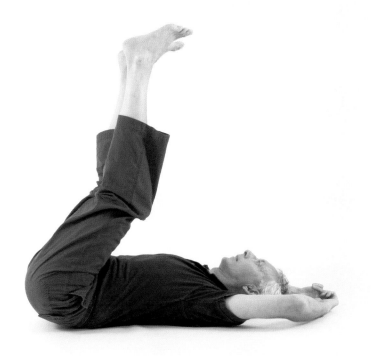

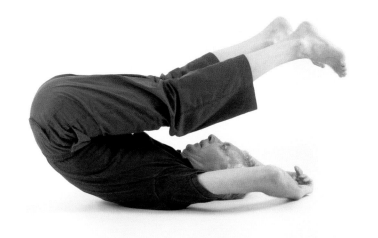

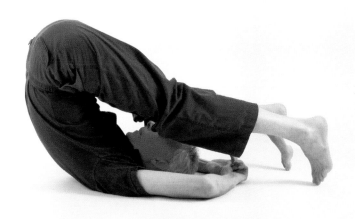

Flexion – a consequence of being upright

Sitting on heels
Vajrasana

The simplest forward bend in this position is the child's pose, or *Pindasana*, and this is where we will start. However before arriving at this simple posture we need first to look at what precedes it. To move into child's pose we first need to be able to sit on our heels. Doing this will quickly expose any problems that live in the ankles or feet. Sitting on the heels demands length in the three vasti quadriceps. These are the quadriceps that just cross the knee, but are not involved in the hip.

This pose also requires length in the dorsi-flexors of the ankle – the tibialis anterior – and the extensors of the toes. If either of these muscle groups are tight the pose will need to be modified in one of several ways.

When the quadriceps are tight, a block can be placed under the sitting bones, so the knees do not have to bend so far. Over time, this can be reduced in height, allowing the quads to lengthen.

When the dorsi-flexors are tight, a roll under the ankle – and not the foot – will take the strain off the foot. Sitting on heels is good preparation for sitting between the heels (*Virasana*), and eventually sitting between the heels and leaning back (*Supta Virasana*), but these poses should not be attempted if props are still required for sitting on the heels.

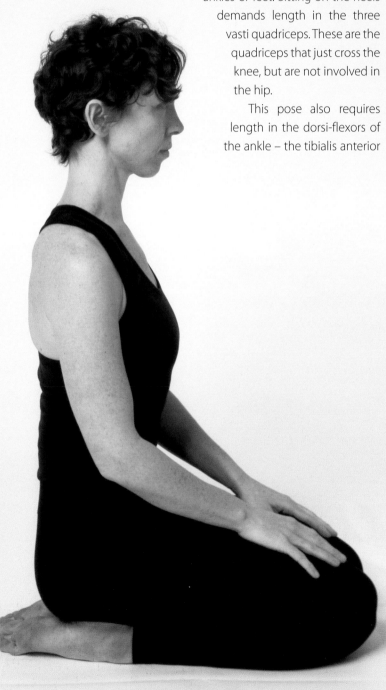

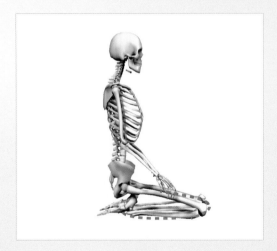

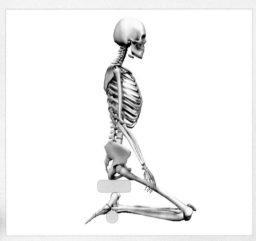

To sit on your heels comfortably, length in the quadriceps and tibialis anterior is required (top inset). When the quadriceps are tight placing a block on the lower leg can be helpful. If tibialis anterior is tight a roll under the ankle is what is needed (lower inset)

Child's pose

Pindasana

The same considerations exist in child's pose as in sitting on heels (*Vajrasana*) in that the quadriceps and ankle dorsi flexors have to lengthen. In child's pose, however, because the body weight is taken forwards, there is less effective weight keeping the hips down. Someone with tight quadriceps might therefore find their hips coming off their heels as they go forward.

The main purpose of child's pose though is flexion of the spine; it is a passive movement and muscles are not involved. What we are interested in here is how the spine curves.

If the lumbar spine is tight and does not forward bend easily, this will often be compensated for by the thoracic spine. If this is the case, it can be useful to lengthen the arms forwards and to widen the knees. As you breathe out, imagine the pelvis settling down on to the heels and the area between the shoulder blades softening and sinking.

In these two pictures (top right), it is fairly apparent that the position of the arms and legs has a significant impact on the arrangement of the spine. In the picture above child pose exaggerates a tendency towards kyphosis in the thoracic spine. By widening the knees and lengthening the arms forwards the upper spine flattens out, a much more useful situation as it encourages an organization that leads away from the habitual pattern.

In these forward bends the knees are bent and so the length of the hamstrings is not a major consideration.

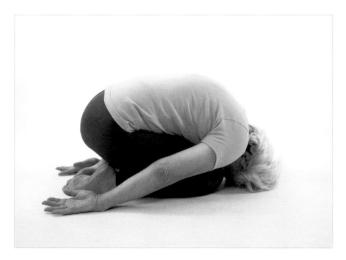

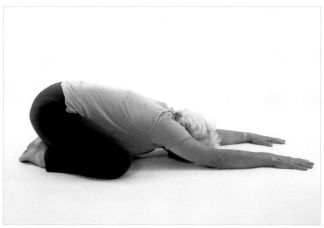

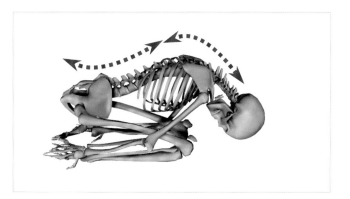

ABOVE
If the lumbar spine is tight and does not forward bend easily it will often be compensated for in the thoracic spine

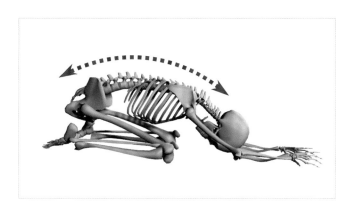

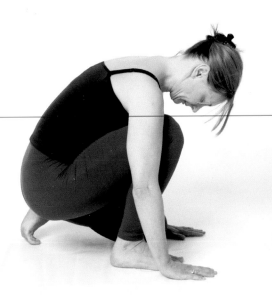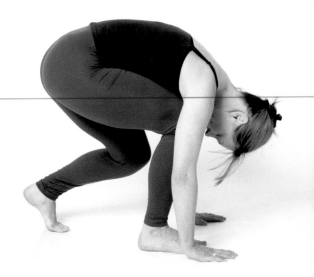

Sprinter's pose

This is a particularly good way of not only progressively lengthening the hamstrings but also bringing mobility into the foot and ankle while, at the same time, informing the nervous system of the very important relationship between the arch of the foot, ankle joint, knee, hip and spine. This is not suitable though for those people with degenerative arthritis in the knees, or inflamed great toe joints.

This position starts a little like a sprinter on blocks. The toes of the back foot are tucked under and the hips are sitting on the heels. The body rests completely on the front thigh and the neck is relaxed. From the waist upwards one must be passive; the work is all in the legs.

Keeping the body resting on the thigh, gradually straighten the back leg. All work is being undertaken by the quadriceps; the upper body remains passive. As the back leg straightens, the foot, the ankle and the knee have to work together to organise the movement. The muscles that act over these joints gradually learn a bio-mechanically sound way of working together.

Finally the back leg straightens and the hamstring is lengthened. Throughout this movement, both posterior muscles of the lower leg – the gastrocnemius and the soleus – are stretched. What is particularly important about this movement is the control given to the feet, knees and hips.

The relationship between the arch of the foot, the ankle joint and the knee joint is important and we need to understand it well. If we start at the bottom, we can see that the ankle joint is in reality two joints

The ankle joint itself is a hinge joint that is responsible for most of the planter and dorsiflexion of the foot – the hinge movement between the foot and lower leg. This movement takes place between the tibia and the talus. Below the talus is the subtalar joint, where the talus rests on the calcaneus, or heel bone. This joint is responsible for the action of inversion and eversion (top right). If the subtalar joint is not well balanced, this results in a foot where the arch is either dropped or over lifted, and has long-term implications on the health of the hinge-like joints of the ankle above, and on that of the knee.

The main muscles affecting the balance at the arch of the foot are the tibialis posterior

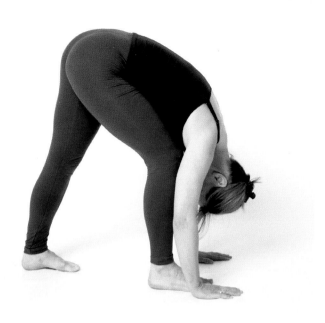

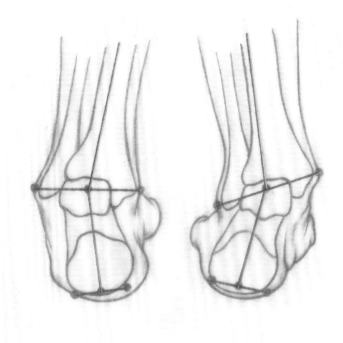

and the peroneus longus. Together these form a kind of sling running under the foot, which supports and balances the arch.

Whenever we practise postures where the feet are on the ground, paying attention to this balance is crucial. Easily the best way to think about this is to imagine weight being taken equally by the inner and outer foot, or to imagine making a perfect footprint on the ground.

It is only when we have addressed the correct balance of the feet, that they, the ankles and the knees have a chance of being well organised.

When we practise yoga we are not only stretching and strengthening muscles. We are, as we have already seen, educating the nervous system in movement. The more we practise, the more we embed, or hardwire, the practised movements into our nervous system. What we do on the mat will slowly impinge on our lives.

It is vital then that we practise sound, positive movements. When we bend our knees we must pay attention to the way our feet meet the floor, ensuring that the knees track, or move forwards, directly over the feet. This way our feet and legs become educated in good biomechanics.

It is only when we have addressed the correct balance of the feet, that they, the ankles and the knees have a chance of being well organised

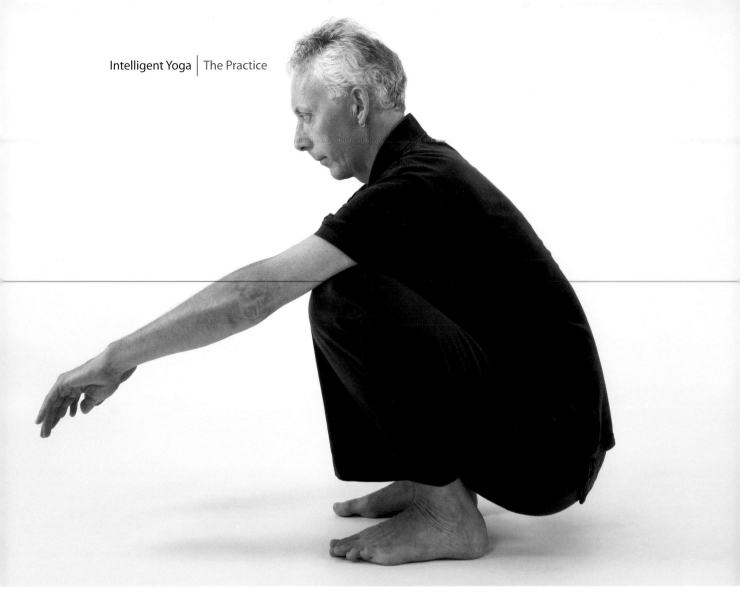

Squatting

One of the important flexion postures bringing the feet and knees into play is squatting. It is a marvellous posture for the lower back and helps to bring good organisation to the muscles of the feet and legs.

Squatting requires good strength in the peroneal muscles and in the quadriceps, as well as a lot of length in the soleus. Squatting is a universal movement; all children squat when they are toddlers, and in many African and Asian cultures people go on squatting into their old age.

In the West, largely because of the use of chairs, we tend to leave this movement behind in childhood. This is a great shame given the many beneficial effects of squatting.

Squatting develops the organisation of the foot and ankle. Like face-down dog pose, it requires length in the Achilles tendon. However, because the knee is bent, it is not the gastrocnemius that lengthens, but rather the deeper soleus. Once the triceps surae

(gastrocnemius and soleus) have reached sufficient length, the heels will stay down in both squatting and face-down dog pose.

Perhaps the most important aspect of squatting is the control of the foot and shin. If the weight can be kept evenly balanced on the base of the big toe and base of the little toe, and the shins kept parallel, the muscles that support the arches of the feet will work appropriately.

This aspect of the pose is vital for practitioners who tend towards flat feet. If the arch support muscles are not working, the arches will collapse and the knees will move towards each other.

When moving both into and out of a squat from standing, the tail bone should drop, keeping length in the lower back. This allows the discs to open up and a gentle flexion curve to run through the spine. To a large extent, one's ability to squat resides in the length of the soleus muscle. However, the relative length of the femur and tibia will also influence the ease with which squatting can be performed.

TOP LEFT
Squatting depends on having our body weight in front of our centre of gravity. To do this, the shin must be able to flex sufficiently at the ankle joint. The soleus muscle (blue) permits this action. If it is tight, the ankle cannot flex sufficiently.

TOP RIGHT
A tighter soleus stops the shin from flexing, and the centre of gravity moves back behind the centre of balance, forcing the person to fall back.

MIDDLE
If we could magically shorten our femurs, then even someone with a tight soleus could squat, because this would bring our centre of gravity forwards. Conversely long femurs would make squatting harder and demand more length in the soleus.

BOTTOM
When we move into squatting the ankle and knee joint act like hinges, with their axes in the horizontal plane (left). If squatting is done carelessly and the joints move out of the horizontal plane (right) problems can develop in the knee.

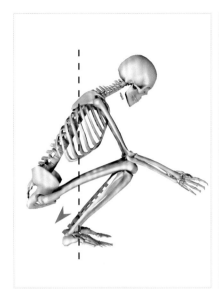
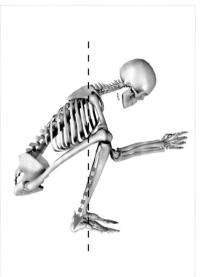
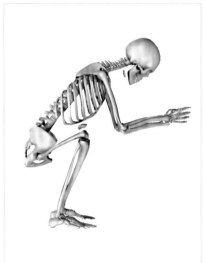
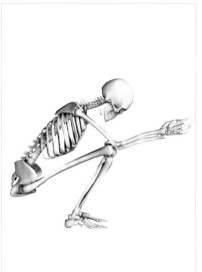
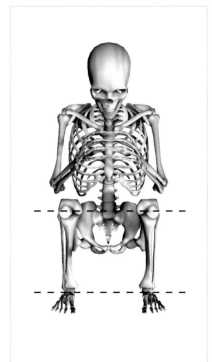
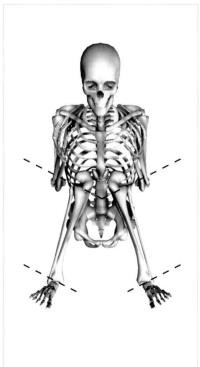

Flexion – a consequence of being upright

Face-down dog pose
Adho Mukha Svanasana

This wonderful posture has many benefits. It lengthens the gastrocnemius and the hamstrings of the leg, and the latissimus dorsi at the shoulder, as well as having the potential to free up the diaphragm and ribs.

When the elbows are brought to the floor, the lengthening of the triceps makes this posture an ideal preparation for a head balance.

If we are trying to enable the respiratory system to find its natural response to posture work, it makes sense not to tighten up around the rib cage and "fix" the muscles of respiration. To this end, how we go into dog pose can be significant. If we start by sitting back on the heels with the toes tucked under and giving weight to the floor through the bones of the arms (rather than pushing back with the arms), the chest and shoulders can relax and breathing can find its own place.

The hips are lifted by the quadriceps and not the arms. It is important not to push through the arms, but to keep the hips as far away from the wrists as possible by drawing the heels towards the ground at the ankles and pulling back from the hips.

In this way, the legs lift the hips while the upper body remains relaxed. The elevated arms will tend to lift the ribs, drawing up the diaphragm and gently releasing tension in it. The belly and pelvic floor will also draw in, following the diaphragm. This is a wonderful example of how the respiratory system is "freed up" as a result of adopting a pose in the most effortless way.

When the hamstrings are tight, however, the sitting bones are pulled down at the back. This forces the lower back to "round out" (top right).

Additionally, if the gastrocnemius is tight, it will be difficult to get the heels down to the floor (upper middle, right).

If the latissimus dorsi is tight and it is difficult to open fully at the shoulders, the upper back will appear rounded, and the weight will tend to move more over the hands (lower middle, right).

As with most flexion poses, it is important to keep the hip flexors from activating unnecessarily. If the psoas tries to pull the body towards the thighs, tension will be experienced both in the groin and the lower back.

It is much better to try and allow the body to fold at the hips softly. But this can only happen when the hamstrings are long enough. In people with very long hamstrings and a lot of openness in the arms, it is possible to take the spine too far through the shoulders, causing the spine to go into compression (bottom right).

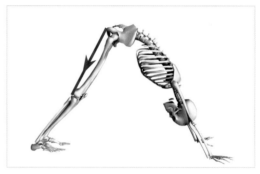

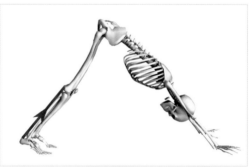

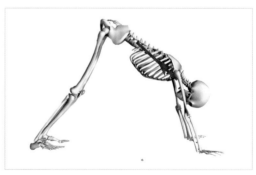

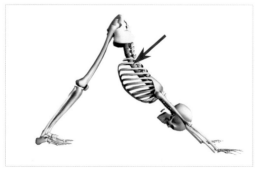

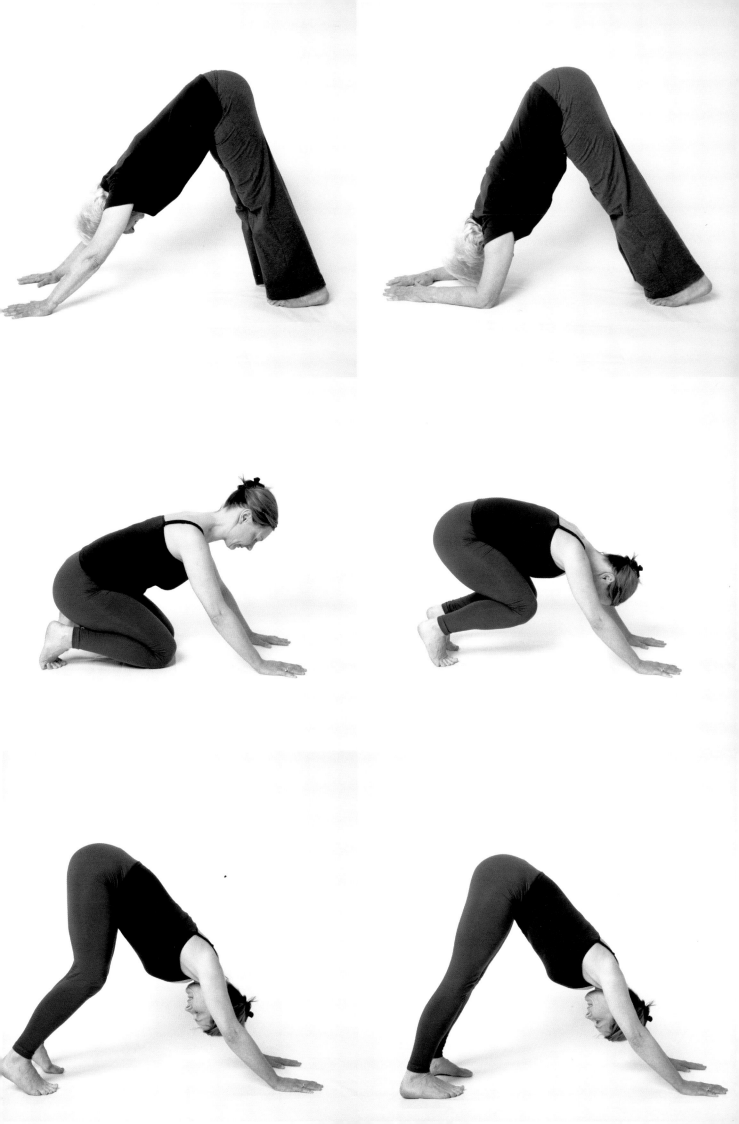

Flexion – a consequence of being upright

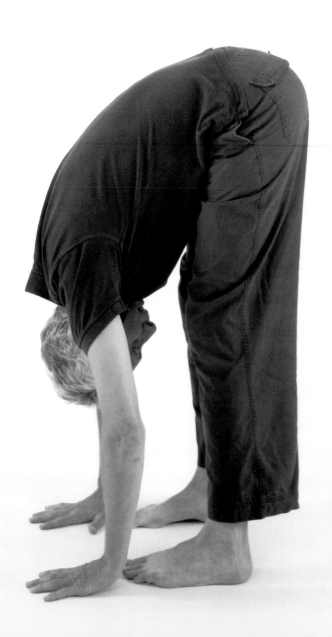

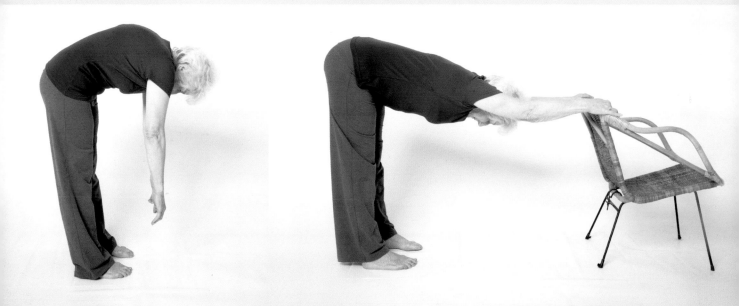

Standing forward bend

Uttanasana

The standing forward bend is a fabulous release for the spine. Gravity acts to open up the discs, taking compression out of those at the bottom of the pile – at the level of L4 and L5.

The upper body weight gives natural traction to the lower spine, and if the upper body can really relax, the arms will tend to elevate the ribs. The weight of the viscera will then fall on to the diaphragm, helping it draw up slightly. The effect of this will be felt in the gentle drawing in of the abdomen and pelvic floor, an echo of Uddiyana Bandha; again it should be noted that this happens naturally, in other words one does not have to do it.

There is a great deal of debate on the safe way to move into a forward bend. It is worth pointing out that forward bending is not dangerous, rather it is a natural function of the spine. In Gracovetsky's book, *The Spinal Engine*, he argues convincingly that the role of the lumbodorsal fascia is to transfer the force generated in the gluteal muscles into the trunk, when the body is coming upright from flexion. He points out that this can only happen when the lumbar spine is flexed because this puts the fascia into stretch and from this situation it can transmit the force of the buttock muscles. However, if the lumbar spine is not flexed the lumbodorsal fascia will slacken off and be unable to deliver the force from the powerful hip extensors.

Some conditions of the spine, such as disc herniations, will make forward bending painful and therefore unadvisable, but the healthy spine should have no problem folding forwards.

If there are problems in the back, then bending the knees is sensible. However, to go forwards with the back straight and stiff as a poker defies common sense. Everywhere you look in nature, movement is rounded and curling; watch a child pick something up from the floor and their back will round, not straighten. This is true of any culture that has to stoop to work, the back rounds because it is safe and less tiring.

When coming into a forward bend from standing, let the back round naturally and, if the knees feel the need to bend, then let them. The same is true when you come back up, rounding the back and softening the knees if necessary will put less strain on the back that coming up flat backed.

When the hamstrings are tight, a forward bend may cause excessive rounding in the upper back in susceptible individuals. This is not helpful because it reinforces the tendency of the upper back to over round anyway. It makes sense in this instance to support the arms, in order that the back can distribute the flexion curve more evenly.

BELOW

In a forward bend the body is supported by large tracts of fascia, ligaments and tendons that include the tendons of the hamstrings, the lumbodorsal fascia and the longitudinal ligaments of the spine

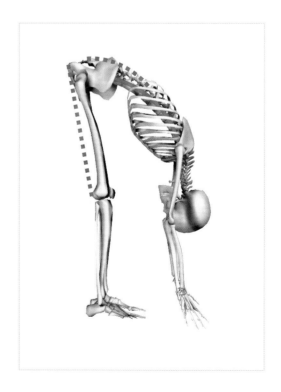

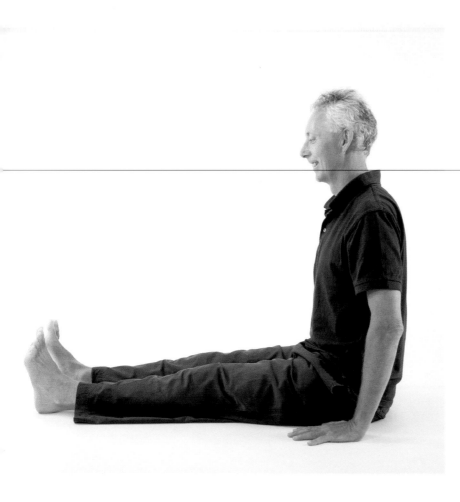

Sitting forward bends

Sitting forward bends are fairly advanced postures, simply because they require significant length in the hamstrings before sitting upright is comfortable. Some yoga practitioners believe that sitting forward bends can be used to lengthen the hamstrings. However, the unhelpful stresses created in the groin make this a poor way of doing so.

Many people find sitting comfortably with their legs straight impossible. Yet it forms the basis of most of the straight-legged sitting postures. Sitting postures can be made easier by varying what we do with the legs.

When the hamstrings are tight they pull on their origin (the sitting bones), pulling the pelvis under and rounding out the back. If we then attempt to sit up straight, our only option is to pull on the iliopsoas against the resistance of the hamstrings. This just reinforces undesirable tension patterns, and we end up sitting with tension in the groin and the back, which is

exhausting. Or, alternatively, the knees will bend.

The easiest way of sitting up straight is by intentionally bending the knees; the hamstrings are then completely slackened and the pelvis is free to sit up or rotate towards a forward bend. To move usefully into a sitting forward bend you must have enough freedom in the hamstrings to be able to have the spine vertical with little or no tension in the iliopsoas.

One solution is to straighten one leg and bend the other. This reduces by half the resistance to forward bending of the pelvis, as only one hamstring is tethering the sitting bones.

Depending on the relative tensions in the hip ligaments of the bent leg, the three one-legged forward bends – the half hero pose, the half cobbler and the half lotus forward bend – are relatively easy or difficult.

To be useful and to enable the spine to release, the body needs to be able to move in front of the gravity line; at this point gravity rather than the psoas can help take the body forwards and downwards.

However, as most of us have experienced at some time, the parts of us that forward bend most easily tend to do too much of the bending. We don't want this to happen because it simply reinforces a poor postural pattern; it is not the upper back that needs to learn to forward bend, but rather the lumbar spine, which is normally held in extension.

I realise that this is a contentious issue, with some authorities arguing that a lumbar curve should be maintained to protect the lumbar spine. To me this doesn't make any sense; a cursory glance at the movement of children, or the squatting postures adopted by many African and Asian adults, show how readily a healthy lumbar spine will flex.

To prevent the upper spine collapsing, we need to keep a sense of slight lift in the upper body so we aren't slumping forwards. This helps prevent the formation of hyper-kyphosis, known colloquially as the dowager's hump, in later life. Sitting forward bends can be useful for developing strength in the posterior supporting muscles of the upper body. With the variations of the leg positions they also provide a good way of freeing up the hip joints.

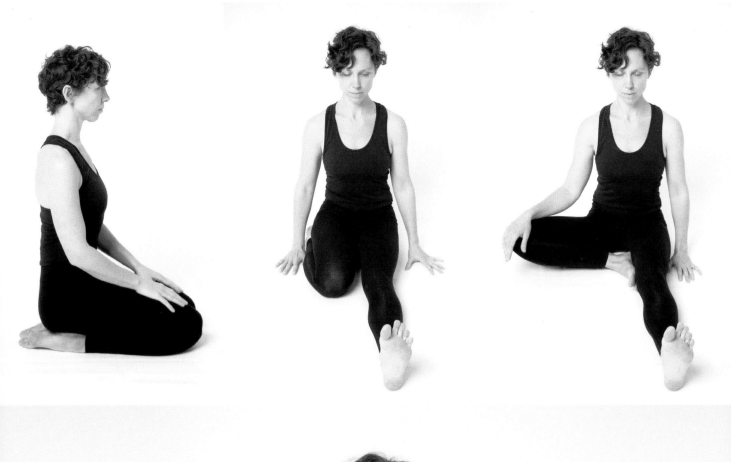
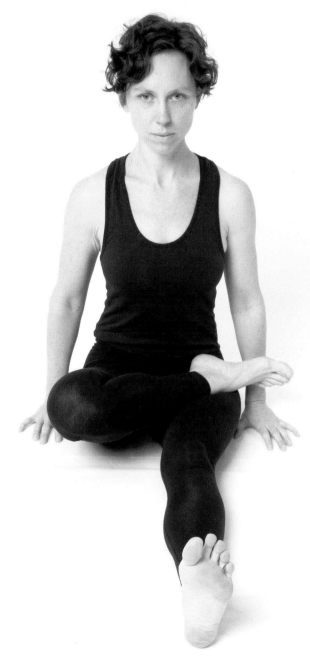

Stepping-forward forward bend

Parsvottonasana

This is a movement into flexion from standing and stepping forward. How far forward one can go depends on the length of the hamstrings.

As there are no other spinal movements in this pose, it can be considered a primary forward bend. Practised regularly it will lengthen the hamstrings on the front leg and the gastrocnemius on the back leg.

As in all forward bends, the emphasis is on moving from the hip and, to some extent, the lumbar spine. What we need to avoid is moving too much from the thoracic spine, as this area tends to move freely that way anyway. Ideally, the hands will rest on the apex of the thoracic curve, and if they maintain their connection, the thoracic spine will tend to remain straightened.

If the hamstrings are tight, there is a tendency to move from the upper spine. This is obviously undesirable as is perpetuates the pattern of the thoracic spine. The idea of flexion is to integrate the curves of the spine so that forward bending is distributed equally throughout the spine, as shown above right.

BELOW
Ideally the curve of the spine should be even as in the top of these two images, however if the hamstrings are tight this tends to exaggerate the curve in the thoracic spine, as shown in the lower image

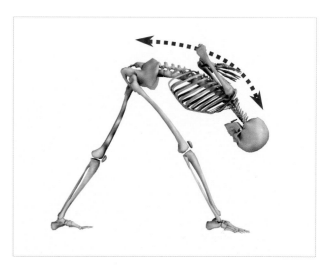

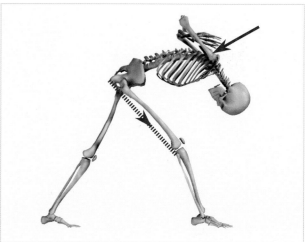

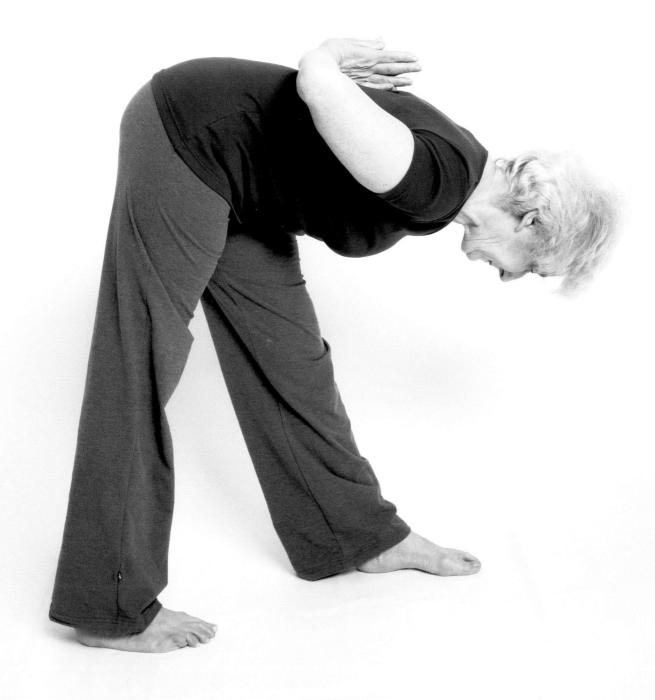

Flexion – a consequence of being upright

ROTATION POSTURES
Twisting for locomotion

It was on becoming bipedal, that our early human ancestor started to employ rotation as a means of locomotion. In the developing child, rotation is the last of the main spinal movements to express itself.

As soon as a baby realises it can twist or roll over, it will do it with great abandon, as this is the first time it is able to move independently. I remember putting my infant son on the floor in the sitting room then leaving the room to make a cup of tea. On my return, he had gone; it was only a muffled noise from behind the door that alerted me to the fact that he had struck upon a form of locomotion, and had kept going until the door had stopped him.

Yet this is not how adults move around. Rather, we depend on the rotation of the pelvis on the spine, a movement extended usefully by the legs that makes walking and running an efficient means of locomotion. Again we can be grateful to the work of Gracovetsky in showing support for this view. A video he made showing a man born with no legs but walking with a normal gait, is testimony to the role of the spine in walking.

In the upright position the lumbar spine is fairly limited in rotation. Most authorities agree

As soon as a baby realises it can twist or roll over, it will do it with great abandon, as this is the first time it is able to move independently

that, as a whole, is cannot rotate much more than seven to ten degrees. However, research carried out by Farfan in 1973 showed that lumbar intervertebral discs tend to rupture in rotation, which seemed surprising when the lumbar spine wasn't supposed to rotate. It was later established that if the spine was to bend sideways first, far more rotation in the lumbar spine was possible. The danger to the intervertebral disc is, then, not through flexion, but through side-bending and then adding strong rotation.

The thoracic spine on the other hand has facets that permit a great deal of rotation, yet it is encumbered by the ribs, which restrict movement in all directions. It is noticeable though that rotation improves enormously if the rib cage becomes more flexible.

The neck has a good range of rotation, much of it coming from the joint between the atlas and the axis, the first two cervical vertebra.

In yoga, much of the focus in rotation needs to be on the thoracic spine and rib cage. When this area becomes "fixed", we start to ask too much of the other parts of the spine, and so strain can occur.

As yoga practitioners, we are interested in the way the body distributes rotation patterns, as we attempt to make this distribution more even.

In standing poses we come against the problem that if rotation is allowed to travel into the legs, then the knees, ankles and feet find themselves having to deal with forces that they are ill equipped to cope with. In such cases, the idea of constraint is useful, meaning that we consciously stop rotation going further than the spine, by stabilising the legs and not allowing them to get caught up in the pattern of rotation.

In sitting or standing, rotation of the spine

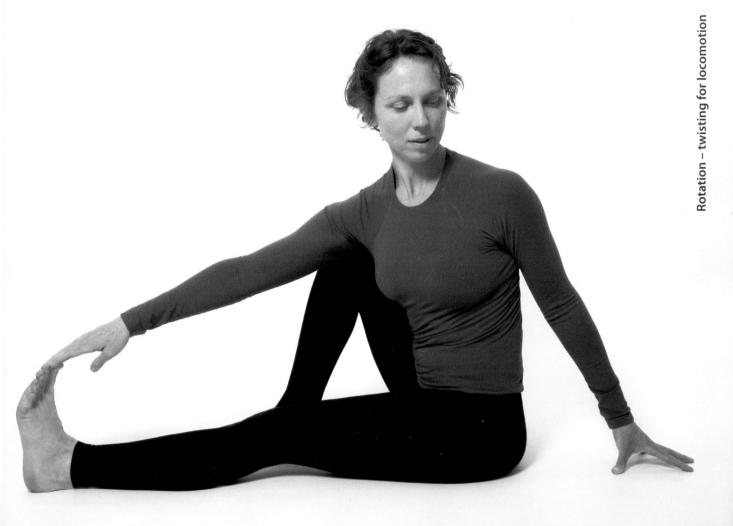

is facilitated by two main muscle groups – the transversospinalis and the internal and external oblique muscles.

These deep muscles do not have much leverage, but seem to be important for maintaining an even distribution of rotation through the spine and stablising one vertebra on another as rotation takes place.

The abdominal muscles on the other hand have a lot of leverage and enable the more powerful global movements of the trunk.

It is the more powerful external and internal obliques that move the rib cage on the pelvis. When twisting to the left while standing, it is the right external obliques and left internal obliques that are engaged, or active.

When the legs are crossed, any movement at the hip joint is removed, so when the knees drop to one side, movement comes from the spine not the hips

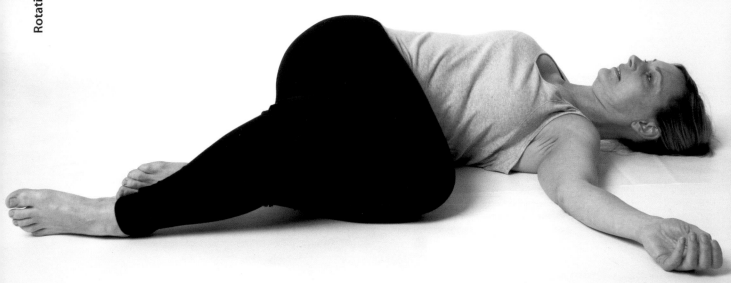

Supine twist

This gentle twist uses gravity acting on the weight of the legs to rotate the spine, and is a good way of loosening up the ribs and thoracic spine.

Because the rib cage is so involved in twists, it is very easy to feel the effect of the breath on the movement. We notice that when we breathe in, the ribs have to expand and the twist undoes a little. When we breathe out and the muscles of inspiration relax, the twist develops a little further.

If our ribs are very stiff two things are noticeable. Firstly, it is difficult to get the shoulder of the extended arm to reach the floor, and secondly, the knees will drift away from each other as the twist develops. This is because when one cannot move in the spine, one will move wherever one can, and this is usually in the ball and socket joint of the hips.

On straightening the legs, the pose becomes stronger, as there is more leverage acting on the pelvis. We may start the pose lying on our back, by dropping the bent legs over to one side; or on our side, by turning the trunk and extending the arm away.

When the legs are crossed, the adduction at the hip is engaged before spinal rotation begins. Therefore when the legs move, this movement originates from the spine rather than from the hip joint. Gravity is the prime mover here, so the posture is better for mobilising the ribs than for strengthening muscles.

When the legs are straightened and kept off the floor this pose becomes strong work for the internal and external obliques, as seen above. Here right external and left internal obliques contract eccentrically to lower the body and legs slowly. The right pectoralis major will also be lengthening.

TOP RIGHT
If the legs are not crossed, much of the movement takes place at the ball and socket joint and little movement occurs at the pelvis

UPPER MIDDLE
When you cross the legs, little movement occurs at the ball and socket joint and the pelvis has to rotate

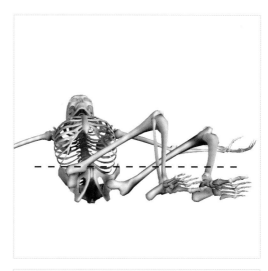

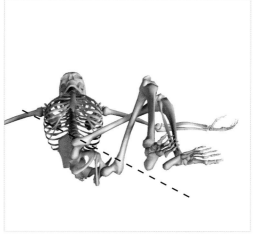

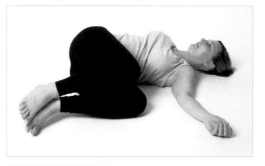

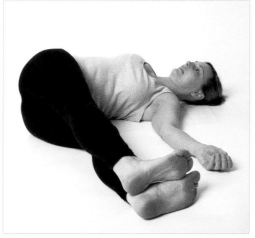

Rotation – twisting for locomotion

Seated twist
Marichyasana one

Most sitting twists are fairly advanced poses simply because they require good length in the hamstrings. As we have already seen in the sitting forward bends, it is difficult to straighten the spine when the hamstrings are tight, because the iliopsoas has to work so hard to keep the spine upright.

In twists, it is helpful if the spine is long. So, if the hamstrings make it impossible to keep the spine tall without tension, it may be better to avoid them or bend the straight leg a little so the back can become straighter.

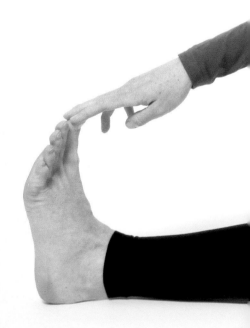

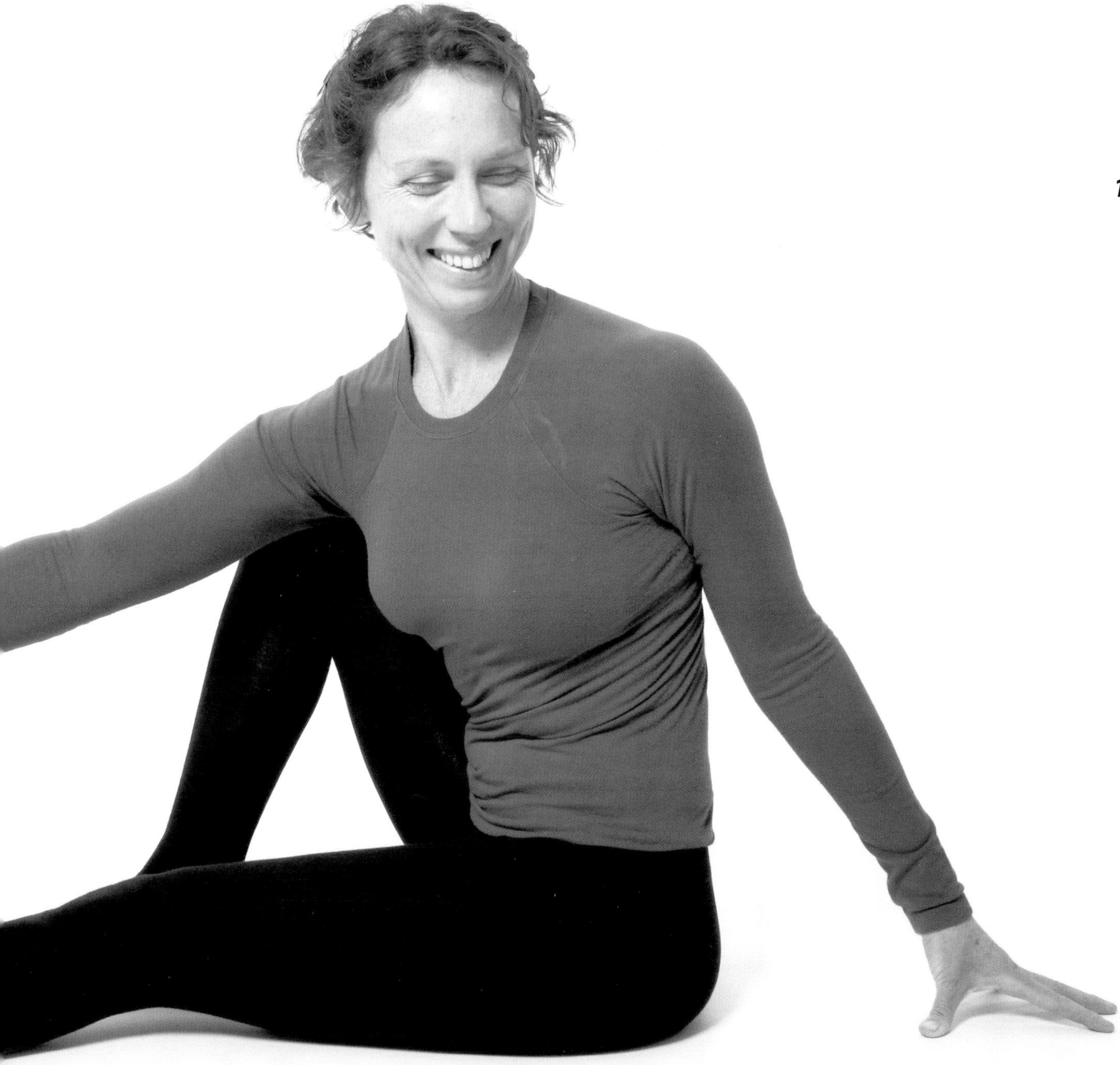

Rotation – twisting for locomotion

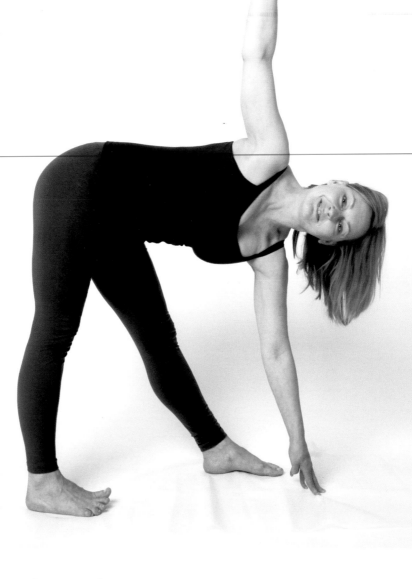

Stepping-forward twist
Trikonasana

This pose is approached in many ways and sometimes there is confusion over its intended results. On occasion it is taught as a sideways lengthening of the spine, and otherwise as a spinal twist.

When taken as a spinal twist, the feet and legs stay parallel and rotation occurs through the spine, particularly the thoracic spine. To allow this to happen, the rib cage has to be free; so using the breath, especially exhalation, is essential for developing the stepping-forward twist. Regular practise will mobilise the ribs.

It is useful to break this pose down into two separate movements. Firstly it is a forward bend, and secondly a twist around the long axis of the spine.

In the first movement flexion is limited by the tension in the hamstrings of the front leg. To stop the chest collapsing downwards the lower trapezius and thoracic erector spinae have to work (far top right). This part of the pose lengthens the hamstrings of the front leg while strengthening the lower trapezius and thoracic erector spinae. The gastrocnemius on the back leg must also lengthen.

In the second part of this movement the internal and external obliques act in unison to rotate the rib cage on the pelvis. The ribs deform their shape to enable the rib cage to revolve, and the thoracic vertebrae rotate on each other along the spine. Deep local muscles maintain the integrity of each vertebra with its neighbour.

It is quite common to substitute movement in the spine for movement in the hips in this pose. When the weight comes onto the back leg, the left hip will drop and the spine will appear to rotate more. A closer reading of the situation reveals that movement is in the ball and socket joint of the hip rather than in the spine.

If the weight is taken more on to the front leg the pelvis rotates the other way, against the direction of the twist, and the twist feels more difficult. We need to understand that if we shift the weight forward and backwards, we move in the hip joint not the spine.

To clarify movement in the spine we need to introduce the idea of constraint; the legs and pelvis need to be stabilised, with the pelvis level. If the pelvis is kept level, then twisting to the left or right should feel equally easy (or difficult).

Thus the stepping forward twist and reverse twist originate from the same base. The difference between the two postures will be felt in the spine rather than in the hips. Perhaps it is worth mentioning here that constraint is useful to bring the attention to areas of stiffness in the body. However, some people are naturally too constrained in their body anyway. In these people it is better to allow some freedom in the movement of their hips.

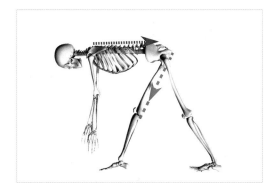

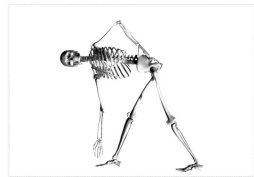

RIGHT
When the weight shifts back, the pelvis rotates rather than the spine

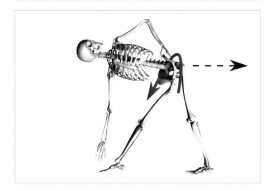

Reverse standing twist

In essence this is the same as the previous twist except that you turn towards the front leg rather than the back one. Because you are twisting the other way, the weight has a tendency to come onto the front foot. This again takes the work away from the spine and into the hips, so the use of constraint is useful here too.

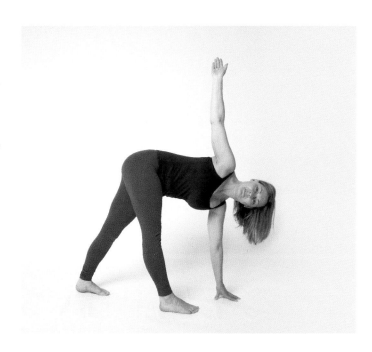

Rotation – twisting for locomotion

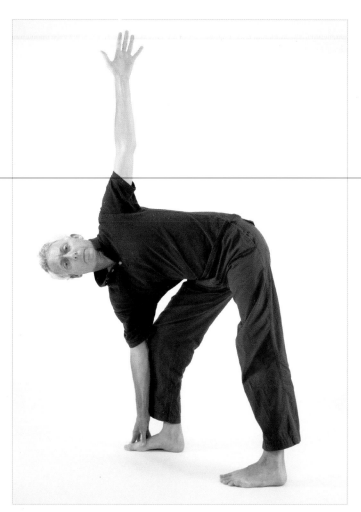

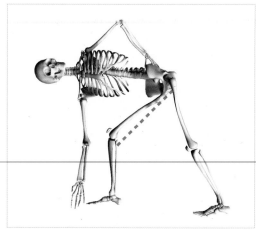

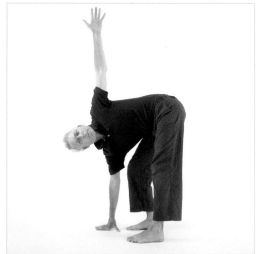

Bent-leg standing twist

Parsvakonasana

This pose is very similar to the stepping forward twist except that the front knee is bent. This has two main effects on the posture. As the knee bends, the hip on that side drops, which takes some of the twist out of the thorax and allows greater freedom in the shoulders for the trunk to widen across the front and back.

Ideally, as the knee bends, the hip on the same side does not move forward. This will then cause the hamstring to lengthen over the bent knee (top right), which takes the stretch out of the tendons behind the knee, and more into the belly of the muscle. It is a very useful way of lengthening the hamstrings.

The more the right hip stays back while the right knee eases forwards, the more the hamstring will lengthen.

Keeping the hip back also keeps the knee in line over the foot, and in so doing protects the integrity of the arch of the foot – and the safety of the knee. The stability and strength of the front leg and foot are the essential basis for this posture.

A standing forward bend, with feet hip width apart, can be used as a basis for a twist (above, bottom right). From a forward bend, one leg is kept straight while the other bends at the knee. Both heels stay down. This makes the pelvis drop on the side of the bent leg, leading the spine into rotation towards the straight leg.

Bending the other leg causes rotation in the opposite direction. Bending one knee then the other at a slow walking pace is very good for freeing up stiff and achy lower backs.

It is important to bear in mind that when the knee bends it should track directly over the midline of the foot, as this reinforces good biomechanics in the foot, ankle and knee.

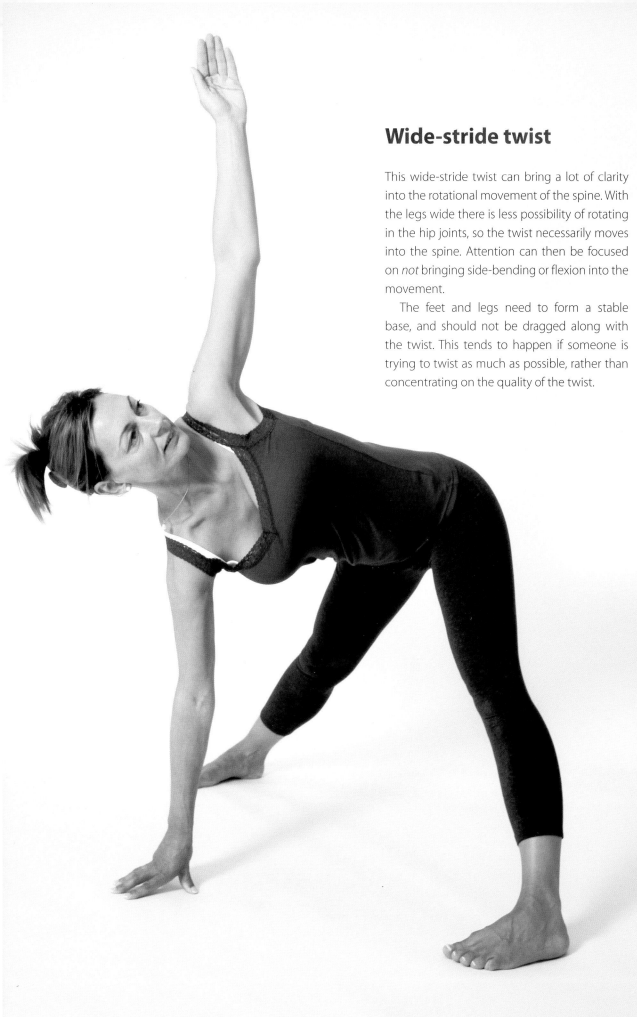

Wide-stride twist

This wide-stride twist can bring a lot of clarity into the rotational movement of the spine. With the legs wide there is less possibility of rotating in the hip joints, so the twist necessarily moves into the spine. Attention can then be focused on *not* bringing side-bending or flexion into the movement.

The feet and legs need to form a stable base, and should not be dragged along with the twist. This tends to happen if someone is trying to twist as much as possible, rather than concentrating on the quality of the twist.

BALANCES AND SITTING POSTURES
Searching for stability

As we have already seen, the patterns of movement involved in yoga are closely related to the evolutionary locomotor muscles of the spine. Yoga postures also take in balances, inversions and more specialised poses that free the hips for sitting.

Balances are particularly useful in helping us understand grounding; how we meet the floor and how steady we become. In the standing balances the feet need to be strong and stable, the upper body free and responsive.

We tend to become tense and stiff when we feel unstable but this is unhelpful – rigid structures topple more easily than responsive ones. The principal concern in balances is to develop poses slowly, steadily and with quiet stability.

Where possible try to imagine weight being transmitted through the bones. These are the structures in the body that transmit forces. When we "find" our bones, muscles can relax and movement becomes smoother and more effortless.

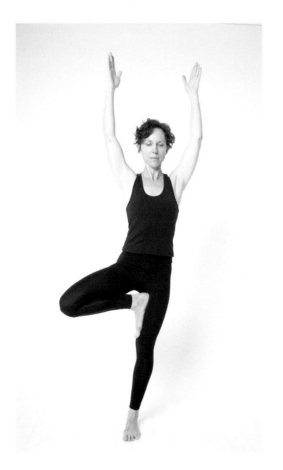

One-foot standing balance
Vrksasana or the tree

The main concern in this pose is to develop a stable, balanced base. The muscles needed to establish such a base are primarily the tibialis posterior and peroneus longus. These muscles balance the subtalar joints, keeping an even pressure on the inner and outer foot.

As much as possible, find your weight down through the bones of the leg, giving this weight to the floor. There is no need, nor is it desirable, to pull up on the kneecaps.

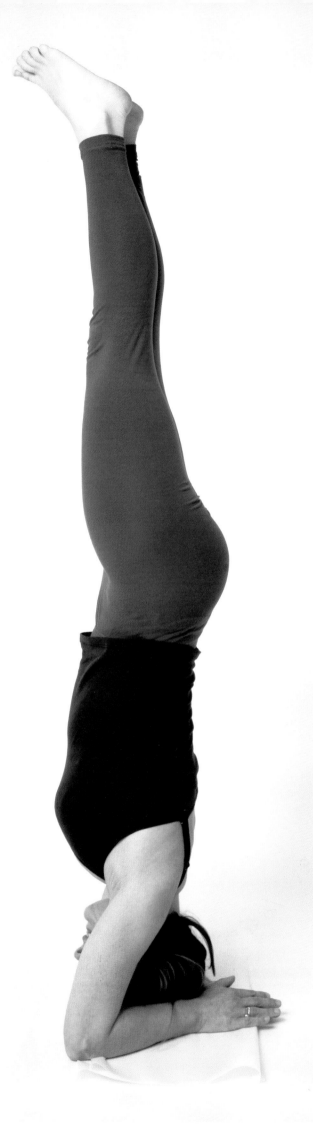

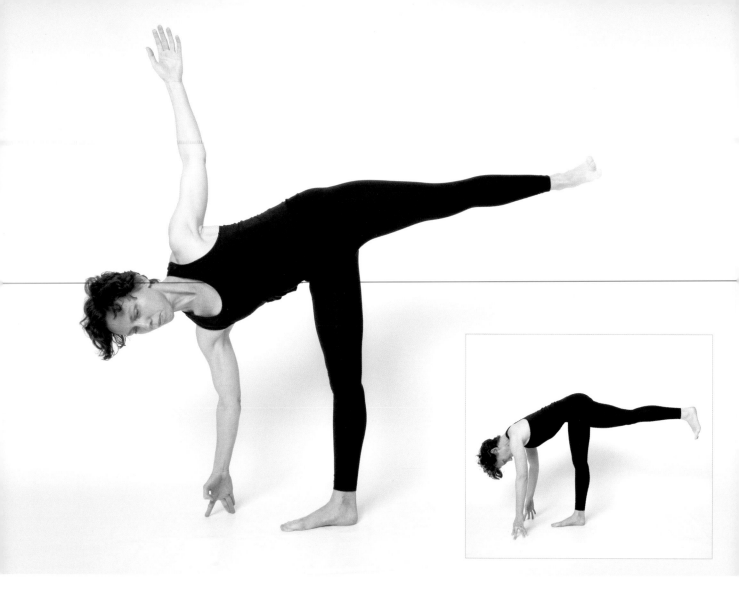

Sideways balance
Ardha Chandrasana or the half moon

Like the tree, this pose requires great stability at the base. It is very easy to allow the arch of the foot to collapse and the knee to roll in, so great attention is needed to keep the weight evenly balanced on the inner and outer edges of the foot (above).

Once stability is achieved, the main action in this pose is around the standing hip joint which moves from adduction through to abduction. However, it is important to become quiet before the hip is lifted. It can be useful, therefore, to spend a few moments in the position shown above before the full pose is attempted

In this pose, the muscles involved in bringing the body from the horizontal position to the abducted position are primarily the tensor fascia latae, and the gluteus medius and minimus shown in red (right). Somewhat surprisingly, the smaller hip rotators such as the piriformis and the obturators act to abduct the body in this position (bottom right).

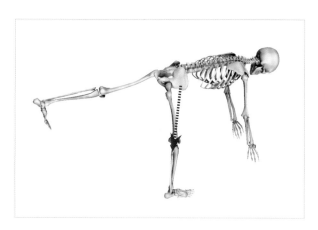

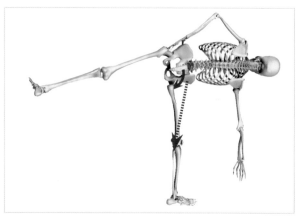

The head balance

Sirsasana

Inverted postures help us fight the effects of gravity. During daily life, fluid flow and the weight of organs are constantly being pulled towards the ground. Although we have wonderful mechanisms at our disposal for responding to gravity, inversions give them a rest: the organs no longer press their weight on the pelvic floor; the venous circulation drains down from the legs, rather than struggling up against gravity; and the weight is taken off the hips and knees.

However I feel the most important aspect of this pose are not the physiological benefits of being upside down, which at best are arguable, but the way it challenges our nervous system. Few other postures in yoga bring up such fear, anticipation and desire as head balance, so it is very difficult to maintain the moment by moment noticing that you need to perform this pose.

It is only when you are able to proceed with complete attention on what you are doing and feeling – rather than what you are anticipating – that this pose becomes safe. It is also worth mentioning here that if we take this perspective on a head balance, it is the quality of movement and grounding that is significant, not how long we stay up.

This pose takes a lot of preparation; the muscles of the shoulder have to lengthen and release, muscles of the neck and spine have to strengthen. When you are quiet and well-grounded the pose should not involve a great deal of effort, the abdomen should be relaxed and drawn gently in – it is not the abdominals

BELOW
This pose developes progressively; stopping at the correct point is critical. Any of the below stages make good stopping points

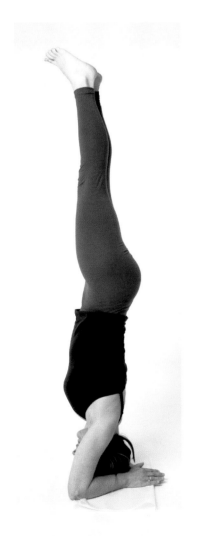

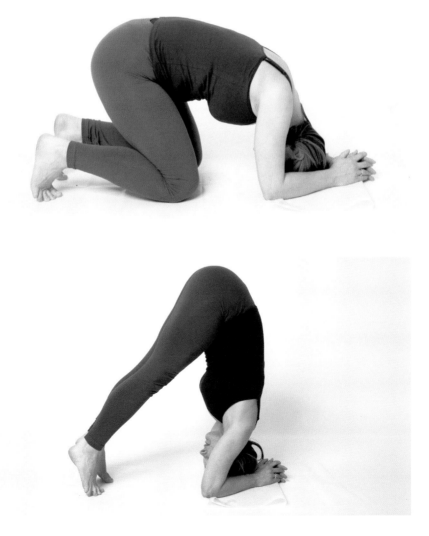

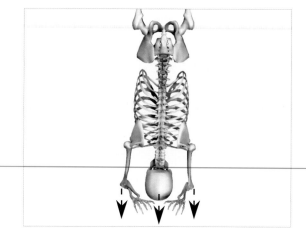

that lift you into the pose.

There are many precursor movements for a head balance. Learning to take the weight into the elbows is an essential first step. Stability in the base and length in the hamstrings and shoulder flexors are necessary before attempting to lift the legs.

The aim of the posture is to give weight to the floor through the elbows and the crown of the head (upper middle right).

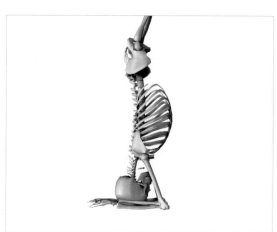

There are three main anatomical considerations when discussing the position of the wrists and arms in a head balance. We need to give the neck maximum length to avoid compression, and we need an arrangement with the arms that maximises the possibility for grounding. The elbows need to be roughly shoulder width apart, which enables the weight to be taken straight through the humerus in a vertical line through the sagittal plane, and provides some freedom in the neck (top right).

It is vital to remember that in a head balance we are not trying to push the head away from the floor. As much as possible we need to think of the weight being transmitted through the upper arms and into the elbows, and through the spine into the skull. Weight comes into the elbows and the head, and the wrists act like stabilisers.

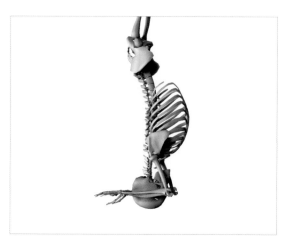

There are a few occasions where the proportions of the arms, head and neck make this version of head balance inadvisable. If the upper arm is comparatively short and the neck is long, as it is in young children, then not enough support can be gained from the arms and too much weight has to come through the head and neck. In this case the three-point head balance is a more suitable variation (lower middle right).

If, on the other hand, the upper arms are comparatively long, the elbows will have to be placed further away from the face, as indicated by the arrow (bottom right).

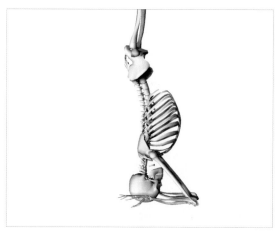

Three-point head balance

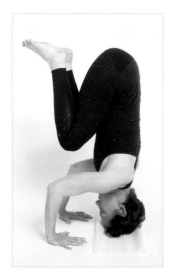

This variation of head balance is initially often preferred, as it tends to give a sense of greater stability. Also many people will have explored this position in childhood. It requires more strength in the arms than the previous head balance, but less flexibility at the shoulders. It appeals particularly to men with strong but stiff shoulders.

Stability in this pose is achieved by keeping the entire hand print firmly on the floor.

In the three-point head balance it is the serratus anterior and pectoralis major that have to work to provide stability for the pose. The pose can be developed by spending time with the knees resting on the elbows. When this feels stable and comfortable the body and legs can be slowly straightened. Raising the legs is done with the extensor muscles of the body, the erector spinae, the gluteals and the hamstrings. The abdominal muscles initially act to stabilise the rib cage on the pelvis.

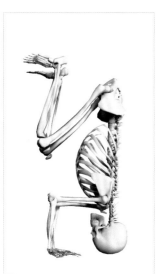

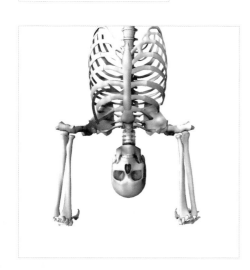

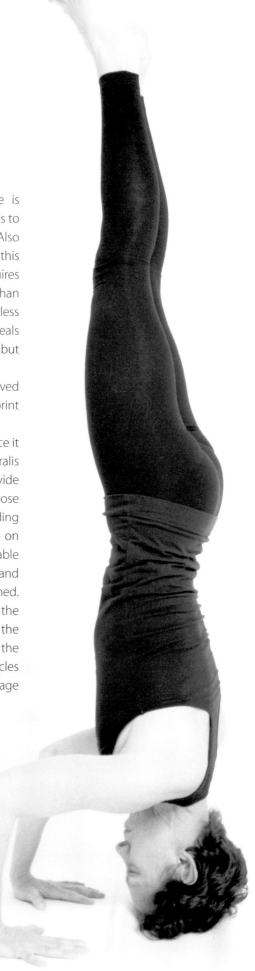

Preparing for the shoulder stand with spinal rolling

Before the shoulder stand is attempted it is very useful to practise these precursor postures. Here the flexion curve of the spine is evenly distributed, reducing stress to the neck muscles. In addition, the spinal extensor muscles are developing the strength needed to maintain the shoulder stand for any length of time.

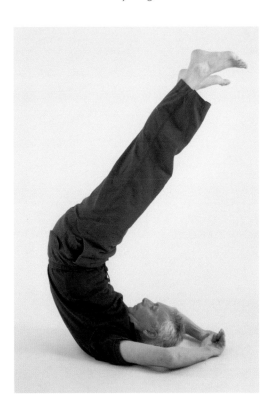

Shoulder stand
Sarvangasana

This is potentially one of the most beneficial of yoga postures but it can take some time to perfect. Apart from the usual benefits of inverted postures on blood flow, the organs and the diaphragm, it has a particularly useful structural effect on a region of the neck that in life often becomes short and tight.

There are many muscles in this powerful area of the body and I will draw attention only to the most significant, namely the fibres of the upper trapezius muscle, the levator scapular, the splenius capitis and the small but important sub occipital muscles. All these muscles run from the back of the skull, traversing the entire neck and inserting either into the scapula, or the upper thoracic spine. Being either extensors of the neck or elevators of the shoulder, these are the muscles we use when we hunch our shoulders and shorten our neck, a common postural habit. The purpose of the shoulder stand is to bring some length back into these often over-used muscles.

In order to maintain a full shoulder stand, we must have enough strength in our back muscles to stop the spine collapsing into a slump, and enough length in the neck muscles so that the body can become more vertical. To be able to get the arms into the best place requires length in the pectoralis minor and the middle fibres of pectoralis major. The latissimus dorsi also needs length as we become more vertical, and although it cannot push the elbows down, once the elbows are rooted by the posterior deltoid, the latissimus can then be used to support the thoracic spine.

Going up into the shoulder stand often presents the novice student with difficulties. This is because of the complex interaction of muscles that are required to lift oneself up off the floor, and the necessary flexibility of the lumbar spine and hips.

As you roll up, you can either pull yourself up with the abdominals, or push yourself up with the arms (posterior deltoid) and to a lesser extent latissimus dorsi. If you always use your arms, the abdominals will not develop the strength to flex the trunk into a balanced pose.

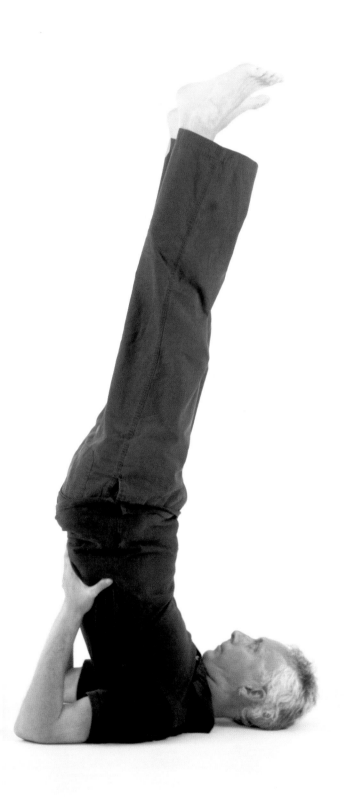

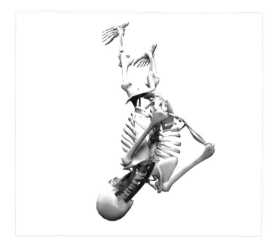

These are the muscles that need to lengthen at the back of the neck and upper thoracic spine, in order that the shoulder stand can become more vertical. Red: upper trapezius, light blue: the sub occipital muscles, dark blue: splenius capitus

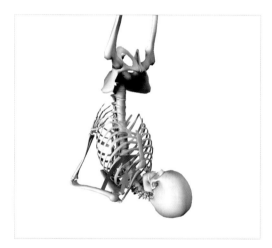

These are the muscles that need to lengthen at the front in order to bring the elbows together and gain support from the floor. Red: pectoralis major, light blue: pectoralis minor

When you roll up into shoulder stand it is the abdominal muscles that get you off the floor. They also have to lift the weight of the legs. The abdominals have to continue to work until the centre of gravity has passed the shoulders; this will be easier if there is enough length in the hamstrings to enable the legs to straighten.

Once the abdominal muscles have lifted the pelvis off the floor, the iliopsoas is no longer required to flex the hip as gravity now does this. If the abdominal muscles are weak, the muscles of arm extension are substituted here. Until the centre of gravity passes the shoulders, it is only the muscles of flexion that are required to work. However, this situation changes.

The shoulder stand is a flexion movement, but one that is moving towards extension. At this stage the flexion curve running through the spine is fairly evenly distributed. As we have seen, rolling up is achieved initially by the abdominal muscles (near right), but once the gravity line is passed, the abdominals are no longer needed and can therefore relax. The spinal extensors are required to straighten the body from this point (far right).

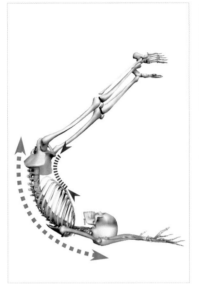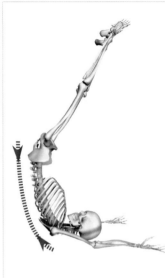

As the extensors straighten the body, the flexion curve reduces in the lumbars and lower thoracic spine, and becomes stronger in the upper thoracic and the cervical spine. The limiting factor will now be the length of the muscles at the back of the neck. It is very important not to over stretch the back of the neck and there is no particular value in the body being vertical. In fact, it is possible to overstretch the facet joint ligaments if verticality is pursued to vigorously.

With the arms over the head it is unlikely that the neck will be strained. However, if the arms are used to push oneself into a more vertical position, the neck muscles can be over-stretched. Care is needed, then, when using the arms for support.

As nearly all practitoners are still slightly in flexion in the shoulder stand, and the tendency is to fall into further flexion, we can see that the posture is maintained by the muscles of extension – the hamstrings, gluteals, erector spinae and latissimus dorsi.

If these muscles are weak, there is a tendency to rest on the arms. If this becomes a habit the back muscles will not strengthen sufficiently to support the pose adequately. Only if you can get perfectly straight can these muscles then relax; but you can only get straight when the muscles of the back of the neck have lengthened sufficiently. In many people this may simply be unadvisable, particularly if the position is going to be sustained.

Some systems of yoga advocate the use of blocks for the shoulders and arms. This takes the stretch out of the neck and enables the student to get the spine more vertical. If becoming vertical is your prime objective, then blocks will help. If, however, you are more concerned with bringing length into the sub occipital region, then avoid using blocks. It should be added though that some padding under the neck and shoulders is advisable if you are working on a hard floor.

One of the worst scenarios for the shoulder stand is when the body is heaved into position using momentum, and the position is then held by collapsing back onto the hands and arms, In this case no muscles work to support the body and the neck risks injury during the heave.

Table pose

Purvottanasana

This is another useful pose to practise in order to help develop the shoulder stand. It strengthens the extensor muscles of the body, particularly the gluteal's and spinal extensors, but it also brings the arms into the position required for the shoulder stand. It is particularly helpful for those people who find it difficult to ground the elbows in shoulder stand.

If the hips can be lifted high enough, the head can drop back, helping bring the upper spine into extension (upper middle right). This should only be attempted if the trunk is horizontal or higher than the thighs, otherwise one risks compression in the neck. In table pose the gluteus maximus provides most of the power to lift the hips, and has to overcome body weight and tension in the hip flexors (lower middle right). If the hips can be lifted high enough, taking the head back can mobilise that very stiff area in the upper thoracic spine. If resistance from the hip flexors and body weight is more than the gluteus can overcome, the hips will not be lifted high enough, and then taking the head back can be dangerous because of compression at the sub occiput (middle right).

If you are comfortable in this position, you can then try straightening the legs (bottom right). This classical version of the pose, with the legs extended, makes it harder to keep the hips high because more extension is required at the hip joint. In this picture the hands point away from the feet, but it is good practice to turn the hands and arms towards the feet sometimes, and on other occasions out to the sides. This puts the rotator muscles of the shoulders through their full range of movement.

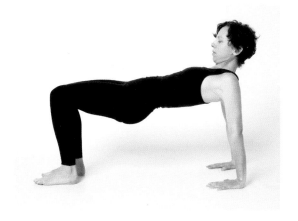

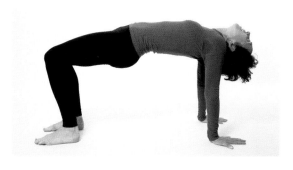

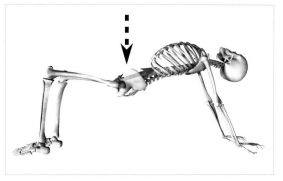

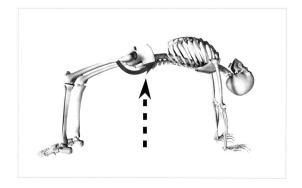

In table pose the gluteus maximus provides most of the power to lift the hips

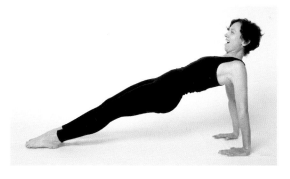

its main benefit is in the strengthening of the front trunk muscles – the abdominals, the rectus and the obliques.

Plank pose

Kumbhakasana

Although this posture is often described as an arm and shoulder strengthener, which to some extent it is, its main benefit is in the strengthening of the front trunk muscles – the abdominals, the rectus and the obliques. These are the muscles needed to resist gravitational sag. The shoulder blades are stabilised by the pectoralis minor, serratus anterior and the rhomboids. Some activity in the gluteals and hamstrings may be necessary to keep the tailbone anchored.

Side plank pose
Vasisthasana

When the pose is turned on its side, the difficulty is still to resist gravity; the underside muscles are now the active ones. In the waist, these are the internal and external obliques, as well as the quadratus lumborum. The hip will be stabilised by the gluteus medius, and the lower leg will find support from the tensor fasciae latae. In both postures the organisation of the arm is important; ideally it should form a right angle with the trunk as this provides the most efficient bony support for the body and will reduce effort somewhat.

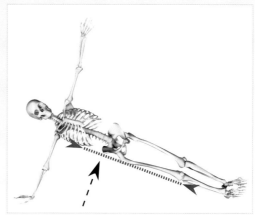

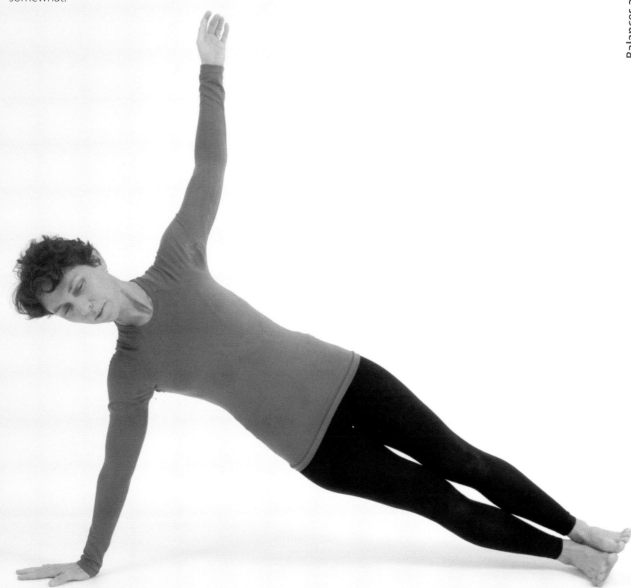

Sitting and the hip joints

To be able to sit comfortably, the hip joints need a lot of freedom. Restriction at the hips comes both from muscles and ligaments. In the practised yogi, the restrictions are usually to do with ligaments. In the novice, muscles are probably the issue.

The hip joint is a ball and socket joint and can therefore move in any direction. However, brief experimentation will quickly assure you that the freedom of movement in all directions is not equal. Some of this inequality of movement is down to the muscles over the hip joint, but perhaps as much, if not more, can be attributed to the hip ligaments.

The hip ligaments

The hip ligaments form a continuous structure completely enclosing the hip joint. For the sake of clarity they are usually divided into three components: the ischiofemoral ligament, the iliofemoral ligament and the pubofemoral ligament. In terms of movement they all share two common attributes; firstly they all tighten up when the hip joint is taken into extension, and secondly they all slacken off when the all-fours position is assumed.

The ischiofemoral ligament

Restriction of movement occurs when any part of the hip ligaments tighten. The ischiofemoral ligament tightens significantly in two planes – medial rotation and abduction.

In yoga, abduction is rarely limited by the ligaments, yet internal/medial rotation is. There are not many postures demanding much internal rotation, only a few sitting poses. Hero pose requires a small degree of internal rotation of the thigh, as does the sitting variation shown below. Both of

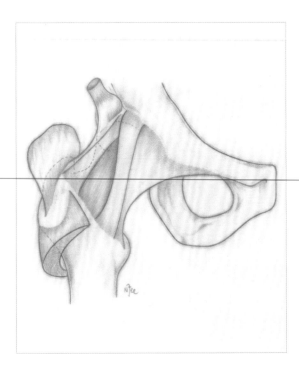

To be able to sit comfortably, the hip joints need a lot of freedom

BELOW

In the picture on the left a considerable degree of internal rotation is necessary in the right hip if both sitting bones are to remain in contact with the floor. If the ischiofemoral ligament is tight, the right sitting bone will be lifted off the floor, as shown below right

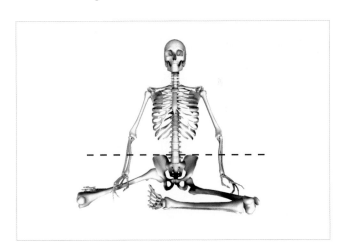

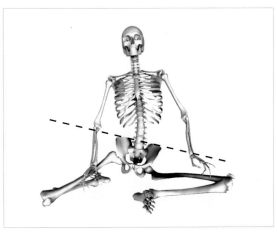

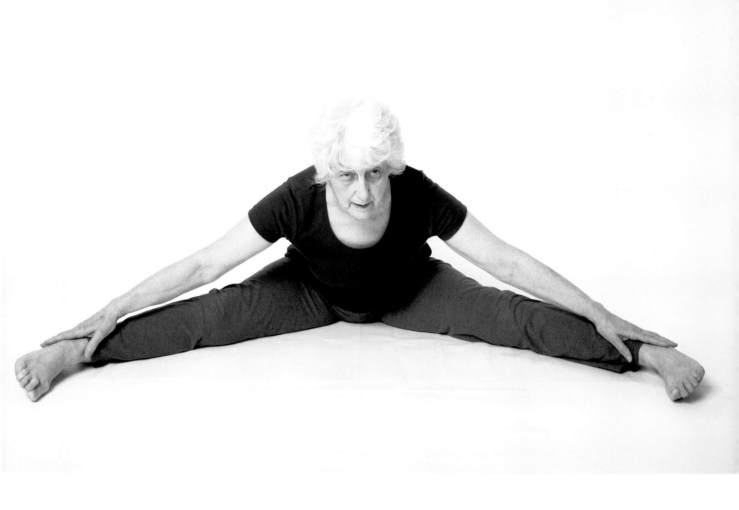

these postures demand a certain amount of internal rotation of the thigh.

Perhaps the more common observation of the hip ischiofemoral ligament is when it is relatively lax; such people can rotate their legs inwards a great deal, even in wide-legged sitting (above).

The iliofemoral ligament

The iliofemoral ligament winds around the front of the hip joint. Its main function is to check extension at the hip. In this it acts identically to the iliopsoas muscle, and it is often difficult to decide whether it is the muscle or the ligament that restricts this function. What is essential to recognise is that once full extension at the hip has been reached, further extension of the leg will bring the pelvis with it, causing exaggeration of the lumbar lordosis and, as a result, compression of the lumbar spine.

A degree of length in this ligament is necessary, both for ease and freedom in upright standing and for improving back bends. When shortness remains in the iliofemoral ligament, back bends tend to compromise the lumbar spine. It is worth noting that this ligament has had to make considerable adaptation to the upright position, both in the evolutionary sense and in the life of the individual. If this process is not completed, it is impossible to fully lengthen the spine in the upright position.

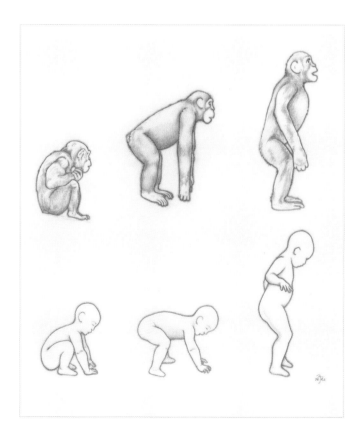

When the iliofemoral ligaments are tight, the pelvis is tipped forward when standing or lying with the legs long (bottom left). It is all but impossible to drop the tail bone and lengthen the lumbar spine. In fact, it is largely tension in this ligament that is responsible for the lumbar lordosis when the legs are long. Any back bends attempted from this position will potentially cause the lumbar spine to compress and possibly risk injury. Until sufficient length in the front of the hip has been obtained, the deeper back bends are probably best avoided.

It is dangerous to talk about "norms", but a rough rule of thumb is that when standing, the asis anterior superior iliac spine (the hip bone) should lie vertically above the pubic bone.

It is also true that the upper fibres of the iliofemoral ligament tighten somewhat during external rotation, so tension in this ligament may cause some difficulty in poses such as the lying version of the cobbler.

Until sufficient length in the front of the hip has been obtained, the deeper back bends are probably best avoided

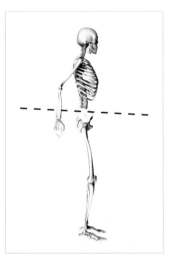

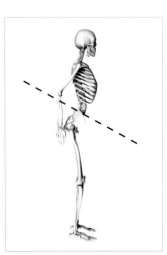

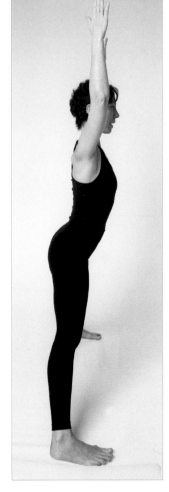

The pubofemoral ligament

The pubofemoral ligament forms the lowest part of the hip ligaments and is perhaps the most significant from a yoga perspective. This is because the pubofemoral ligament tightens up on external rotation and abduction, two commonly performed movements in sitting asanas. Cobbler pose (*Baddha Konasana*) is perhaps the most extreme of these. However, flexion of the hip will tend to slacken this ligament, as it does to all hip ligaments, so to some extent the effects of abduction and external rotation are ameliorated. In standing with a wide stride, the pubofemoral ligament tends to pull the pelvis forward, increasing the lumbar lordosis (near left). This may also be caused by tension in the adductor muscles, particularly the pectineus. If external rotation of the legs markedly increases the lordosis, the tension is probably ligamentous. Muscular tension will also be felt down the inside of the thigh, as far as the knee. If it is just the ligament, then you are more likely to feel it in the groin.

It is difficult to say with certainty when a ligament is providing resistance to movement and when a muscle is. Two things may be helpful to remember when trying to decide. In the hip at least we can say that ligament resistance will be felt close to the joint, whereas muscular resistance is usually felt further away from it. Also, if you practise regularly, with time you are likely to overcome most muscular resistance. What resistance remains then is probably the ligaments. It is also worth remembering that ligaments create stability: forcing ligaments to stretch is not a good idea.

Wide-legged sitting
Upavistha Konasana

To sit comfortably in this posture you need length in the hamstrings, the adductors and the pubofemoral ligament. If the adductors or the pubofemoral ligament are tight it will be difficult to take the legs wide enough apart. If the hamstrings or the longest adductor (adductor magnus) are tight, then the pelvis will be pulled under and the back will round out.

Because adductor magnus originate on the lower part of the ischiopubic ramus, this will tend to pull the underside of the pelvis forward as the legs are widened. It is similar to the effect that tight hamstrings have in the sitting-forward bend. The difference is that the hamstrings are slightly slackened off as the legs are spread. So unless they are quite tight, the hamstrings tend not to be the major problem in this pose.

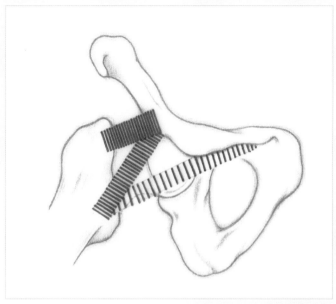

The pubofemoral ligament stretches when the leg is abducted

Balances and sitting postures

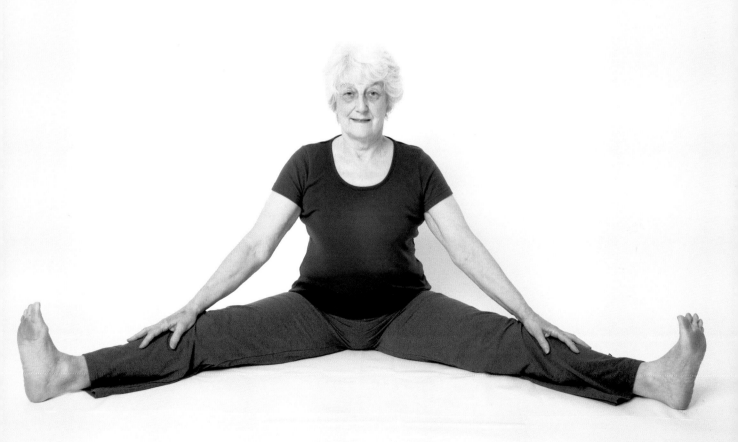

Cobbler pose
Baddha Konasana or bound angle pose

Bending the legs increases abduction of the legs and adds considerable external rotation of the femur. This causes further stretching of the adductor magnus, which may cause a posterior tilt to the pelvis, pulling the tailbone down, and therefore, causing the rounded back so commonly seen in this pose.

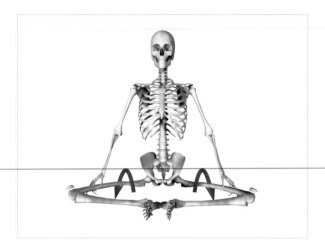

150

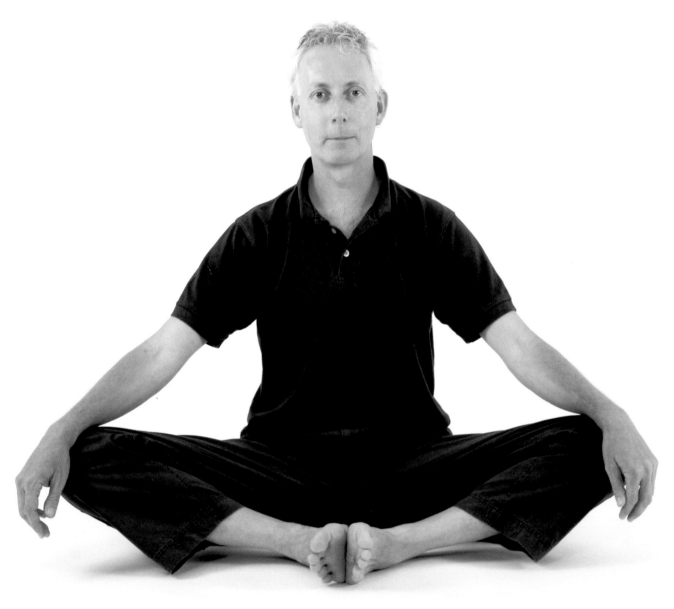

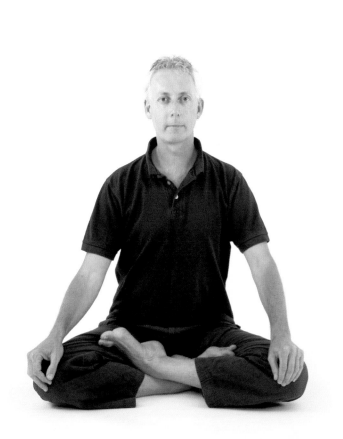

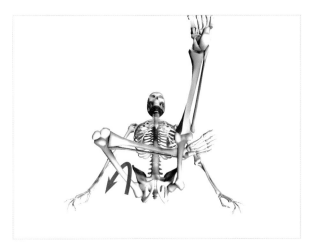

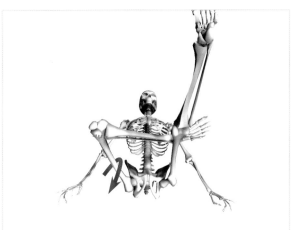

Cross-legged sitting

Padmasana, lotus or half lotus

The lotus or half lotus requires further external rotation of the femur, but the thighs are closer together than in cobbler. It is, therefore, unlikely that the adductors restrict this movement. Because of the extreme external rotation required, the probable restriction to this posture is the pubofemoral ligament.

If the hip is unable to rotate externally, then trying to force the foot into position will cause strain on the lateral collateral ligaments of the knee. This is a common cause of knee problems in yoga and meditation students. Most cross-legged postures will put some stretch on the lateral collateral ligaments, which in itself is not a problem as a degree of elasticity here is desirable.

Lotus position demands more external rotation of the thigh than other sitting poses. Some adduction of the lower leg on the thigh is inevitable and causes some stretch of the lateral collateral ligaments. If the thigh is restricted in external rotation the lower leg will have to be adducted more to get the foot into place and this is when overstretch injuries to the ligaments are possible (above lower right).

Balances and sitting postures

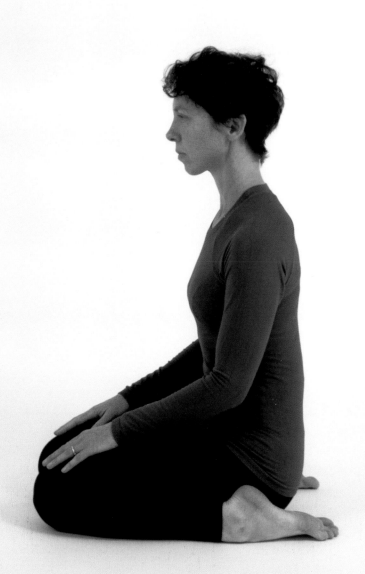

Sitting between the heels

Virasana or hero pose

This posture is a development from sitting on heels (*Vajrasana*). Sitting on heels is good preparation for hero pose and eventually for supine hero pose (*Supta Virasana*), but neither of these should be attempted if you still require props when sitting on your heels.

Sitting between your heels should only be attempted if the knees are healthy and it can be done with ease. The posture involves widening the space between the feet and sitting on the floor between them.

This necessitates some internal rotation of the thigh and abduction of the lower leg at the knee. The action at the knee causes some lengthening of the inner compartment of the knee, which needs to be balanced with the lengthening of the outer compartment, by doing some cross-legged poses.

There is potential danger to the knee if the mechanics are not fully understood. A large part of taking the feet out is done by the internal rotation of the femur, in the picture (top right) there is no strain on the knees.

Sitting on heels ensures that the quadriceps and tibialis anterior have enough length before hero pose should be attempted. Gradually the feet can be widened and the hips lowered towards the floor which, slowly lengthens the medial compartment of the knee . If the knees become uncomfortable, it is important to sit on a block.

As the knee bends there is an opening up of the inside of the knee (bottom right). This stretches the medial collateral ligament. A certain amount of "give" in these ligaments is natural for the knee and hero pose can help maintain this. It should be remembered that in hero pose the entire weight of the body can be brought to bear on this ligament, and care must be taken to avoid over-stretching it.

Because hero pose stretches the inner knee, and the lotus and other cross-legged postures stretch the outer knee, these two poses complement each other and help create healthy elasticity in the collateral ligaments of the knee. It should be emphasised though that progress towards these poses needs to be slow and careful. Pain in the knee must never be tolerated when practicing them.

> *Sitting between your heels should only be attempted if the knees are healthy and it can be done with ease*

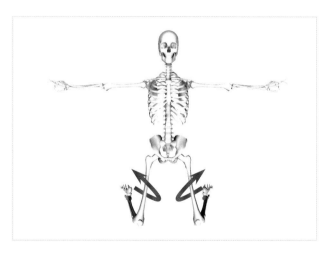

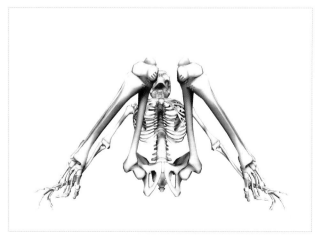

Lying between the heels

Supta Virasana or supine hero pose

Supine hero pose is a significant posture, but is often avoided because of discomfort to the knees or lower back. It is essential to deal with these problems before proceeding with the pose. It is the most efficient posture in terms of stretching the rectus femoris, (the only bi-articular quadricep), a muscle that plays a significant role in balancing the pelvis.

The rectus femoris crosses both the hip joint and the knee joint. When the knee is fully flexed and the hip extended, this muscle is at maximum stretch. If the rectus femoris is tight it will pull on the front of the pelvis causing an anterior tilt. This will lead to compression of the lumbar spine, which is unhelpful, and modification is necessary.

To prevent compression in the lower back, the head and shoulders need to be supported to take the curve out of the lumbars. Failing that, the support of a wall can be equally effective.

The significance of lengthening the rectus femoris becomes apparent when we consider its relation to the mechanics of the pelvis. We must remember that the pelvis rests on the heads of the femurs in freely mobile ball and socket joints. How the pelvis orientates itself depends on the various pulls exerted by muscles and ligaments. From below there are two main groups of muscles that act as restraints to the pelvis: the rectus femoris and the hamstrings.

A relatively tight rectus will contribute to an anterior tilt of the pelvis and, as a result, lumbar compression. In yoga we do a lot of stretching of the the hamstrings but much less so of the rectus. This can lead to imbalance of the muscles that influence the pelvis from below.

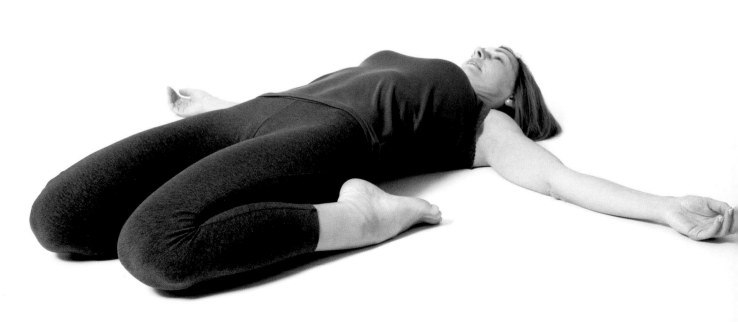

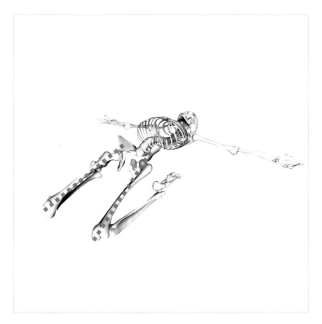

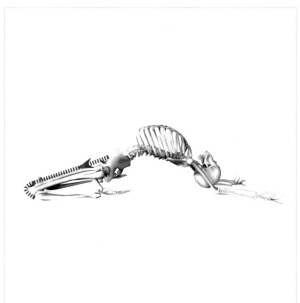

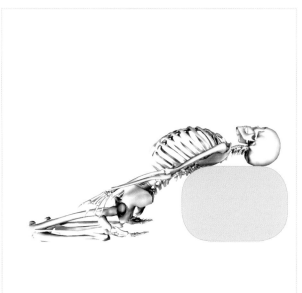

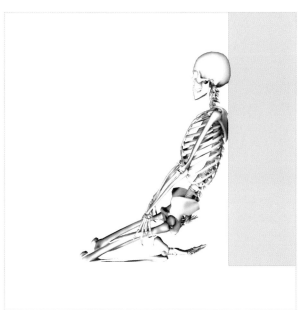

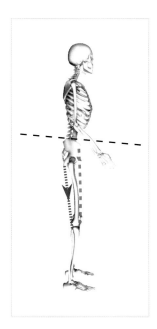

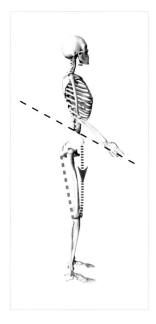

When the rectus femoris is tight, it pulls on the front of the pelvis. If you try to lie back under these circumstances, the lumbar spine will come under compression (top right). If this is the case, you are better supported by a bolster or, failing that, a wall (above left and right). The relative length in the hamstrings and rectus femoris has an influence on the way the pelvis tilts (as shown in both images, left)

In the image on the far left, the hamstrings act to anchor the pelvis from below, helping to keep it level. If the rectus femoris is tight and the hamstrings over-lengthened, the pelvis will be tipped forwards, exacerbating lumbar compression

Legs crossed at the knee

Gomukhasana or cow pose

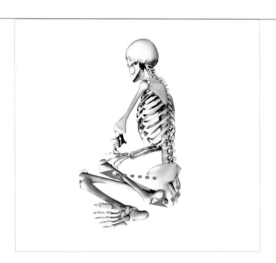

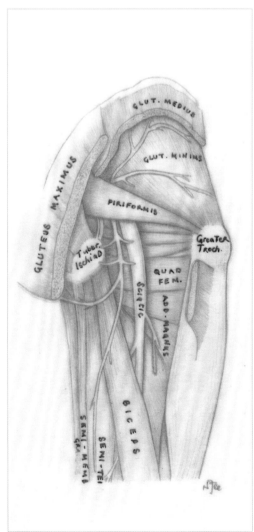

This is an unusual posture because, unlike any other, it asks for adduction of the legs. It is one of the few poses that lengthens the abductor muscles of the leg. There is also some stretch to the piriformis muscle, which is exaggerated by leaning forward. In this pose we are slowly trying to let both sitting bones settle on to the floor.

The tensor fasciae latae is stretched by the adduction of the femur. However, leaning forward will tend to take the stretch off because it adducts both legs. It is also possible that the ischiofemoral ligament provides some resistance in this pose.

The piriformis is another significant little muscle that occasionally causes problems when it is tight. It runs from the sacrum to the greater trochanter of the femur and in standing its main function is to externally rotate the thigh. It shares this job with a few other small external rotators, namely the gemellus, quadratus femoris, and the obturators exturnus and internus.

These muscles can be seen in these posterior cut away views of the pelvis. The significant thing about the piriformis is its relationship to the sciatic nerve, which passes through the space just below the piriformis and above the gemellus superior. In a small percentage of people the nerve passes directly through the piriformis. Tension in this muscle can cause pressure on the sciatic nerve, so learning how to lengthen it can be very helpful. In cow pose these muscles are stretched when you lean forward.

TOP LEFT

Both tensor fasciae latae (long arrow) and piriformis (short arrow) are lengthened in this position

*It is one of the few poses
that lengthens the abductor
muscles of the leg*

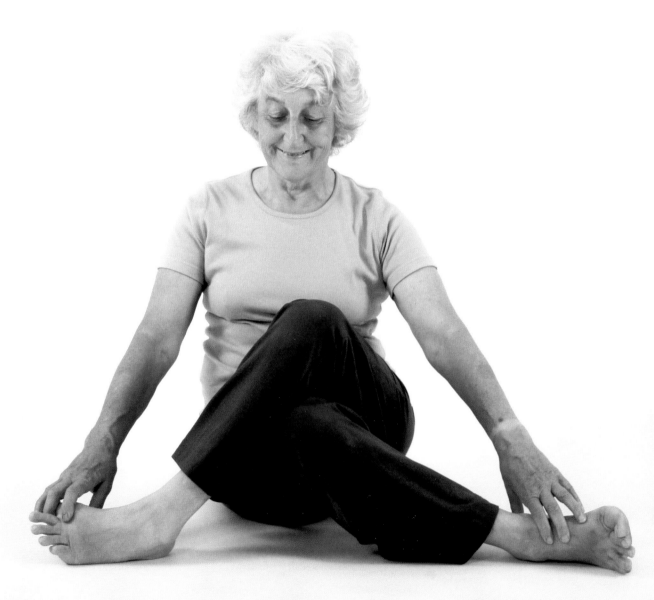

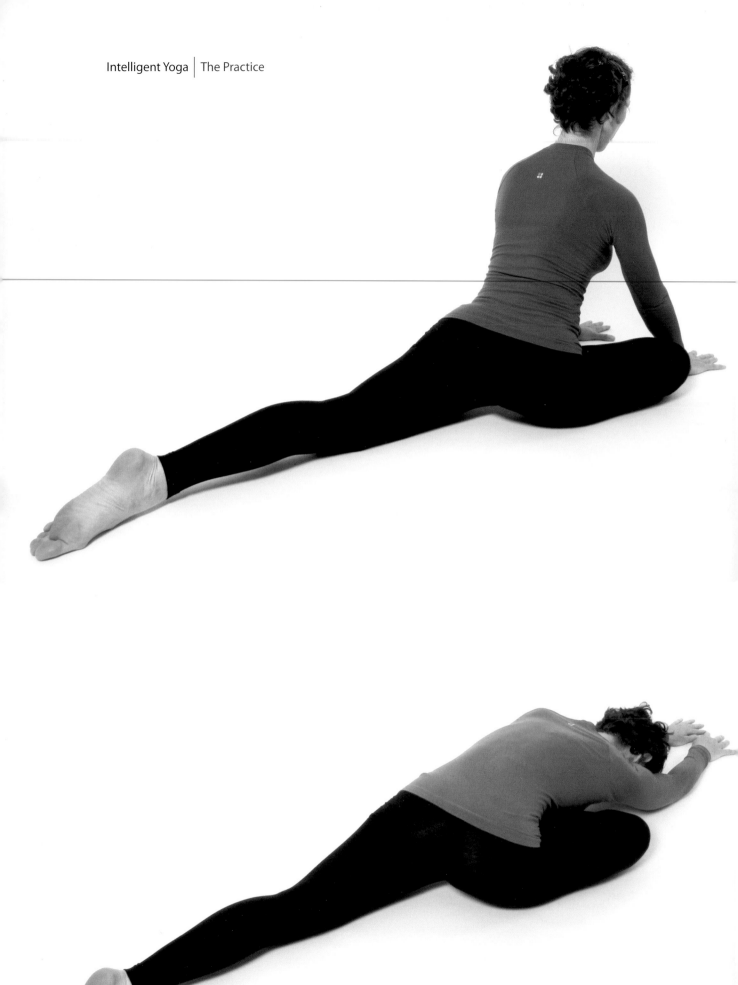

The pigeon
Eka pada raja kapotasana

The preparation for this posture is a movement that addresses tightness in the piriformis. Initially the main concern is to level the hips laterally and allow them to settle down towards the floor. The lower the pelvis drops, the more the stretch on the piriformis.

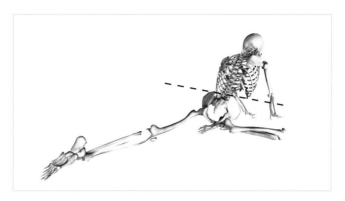

Two aspects of this pose increase the stretch on the piriformis: dropping the opposite hip and externally rotating the right thigh. If the left piriformis is tight it will cause the right hip to lift up (middle right). Dropping the right hip is the primary aim of this part of the pose.

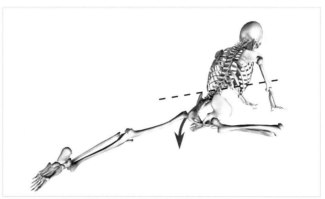

There is some dispute about the position of the front leg. Some teachers like it brought forward to a right angle, others not. It can be seen that, once again, external rotation of the femur is a pre-requisite for bringing the lower leg forward (lower middle left). If you try and bring the leg forward without externally rotating the femur, you risk straining the knee as you would in lotus position; or the right hip will lift, compromising the next part of the pose. Therefore for most people it is inadvisable to bring the lower leg forward too much (lower middle right).

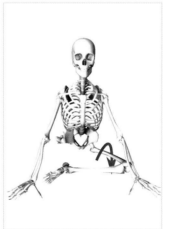 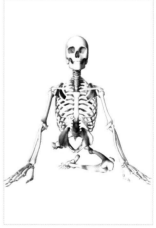

As this pose develops, it turns into a beautiful extension posture. Few people benefit from taking it much further than this, though some can and if they can it can be noted that all the movement will come from the lumbar spine.

At this stage, extension has to develop at the hip of the back leg; the upper back can be fully involved so the extension curve is integrated throughout the spine. The early stages of this posture lengthen the posterior muscles of the hip on the front leg, and the anterior muscles of the hip on the back leg, giving the hip a balanced workout in most of its planes of movement.

Because the front leg is in flexion at the hip the gluteus maximus helps anchor the back of the pelvis down. This is very helpful, as it reduces lumbar compression, making it easier to focus your attention on the movement in the thoracic spine.

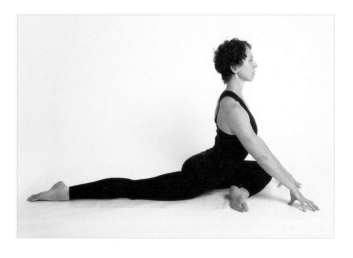

Critique of some modern standing postures

As I mentioned in the opening chapters, yoga has been with us in the West for a good 50 or more years. Posture work has many forms and systems, and it is up to the individual to decide the style that best suits him or her. However there are a few commonly taught postures that, I believe, cause significant joint problems in those who practise them regularly. The chief culprit is the wide-stride warrior pose, or *Virabhadrasana One*.

The first problem to consider is what happens to the knee of the back leg. If this pose is taught with the foot of the back leg turned out by about 30 degrees, and the hip facing forward, two things will inevitably happen, the arch of the foot will collapse, and a rotational force will be put through the knee.

Neither of these is in any way useful, and what happens to the knee is potentially dangerous. The cartilage in the knee does not enjoy rotational forces; in fact repeated rotational stress through the knee can eventually tear the cartilage.

Secondly, we need to look at what is happening in the lower back. When we take a wide stride and turn to face the front leg, the iliopsoas and iliofemoral ligaments are tensioned to their limit. This pulls the pelvis into an anterior tilt, compressing the lumbar spine. The tighter the structures at the front of the hip, the greater the compression on the back of the spine. If the hip is stiff the pelvis cannot come forwards enough and this hip will then be higher than the other one. This will introduce sidebending and rotation into the lower spine while it is under compression – a recipe for disaster (near right top and bottom).

A solution would be to turn the back foot to face forwards. This takes torsion out of the knee and helps the hip come round slightly. But the stride also needs to be narrowed for most people, so that the pelvis and therefore the lumbar spine can be brought into a stress free alignment.

All forward facing poses which involve the back foot being turned out present similar problems for the knees. Most students simply do not have the freedom in their hips to remove strain at the knee. Although I have been taught many variations of these types of poses, nothing solves the problem as well as pointing both hips and feet in the same direction, and perhaps surprisingly, very little if anything is lost in terms of the stretch offered by the posture.

there are a few commonly taught postures that, I believe, cause significant joint problems in those who practise them regularly. The chief culprit is the wide-stride warrior pose

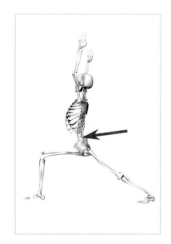

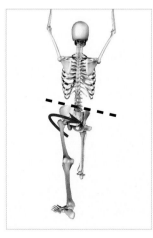

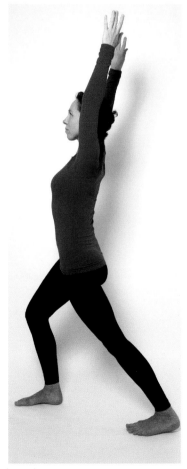

Some forms of stepping-forward twist (*Trikonasana*):

This posture is sometimes taught as a side bend, as though the entire body is in contact with a wall behind it, with the feet turned out to the side. In this case the movement in the spine is pure side-bending.

However, to keep the right hip back, the right knee will inevitably roll inwards, putting an unnecessary and unhelpful rotational force through the knee (top right). To make the side bend safe for the knee it makes much more sense to point both the feet, both the knees and the spine forwards (upper middle right).

Some teachers allow the hip of the back left to drift forwards and the hip of the front leg to drop. This reduces rotation, and therefore, stress on the knee joint, making the posture safe. Now, however, the pose is merely a mild twist in the spine and a gentle stretch in the leg; it becomes pointless.

It is sometimes suggested that the arm should stretch sideways while the hip drops, allowing the waist to lengthen This may be fine for people with very flexible hips, but those with stiffer hips risk injury to the lower back.

When the spine is asked to lengthen sideways, the movement can be accommodated to some extent by the individual joints and discs of the spine. At some point, though, the sideways movement meets the lumbosacral and sacroiliac joints, which are relatively fixed in place.

The force then becomes a shearing force where the spine meets the sacrum (bottom right). Practised infrequently this probably is not a problem. If on the other hand you practise this move diligently, instability at the lumbosacral or sacroiliac joint can follow, creating difficult problems to resolve.

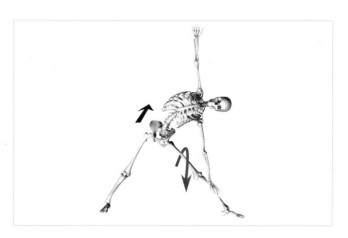

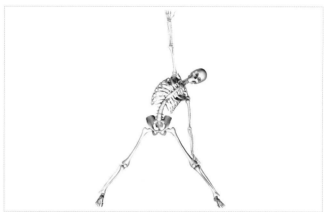

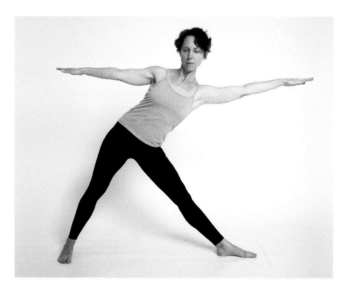

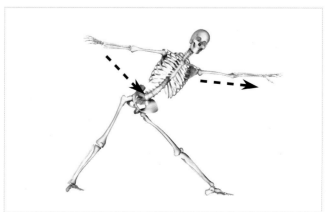

PRACTICE AS A ROUTE TO ENQUIRY
Noticing habits, developing choice

If we take yoga seriously we will practise a lot. It makes sense, then, that what we practise has a positive impact on the body. I have explained already why I think working with the locomotor patterns is important. I would argue similarly for the legs: nearly all of the standing poses can be taught with the feet parallel and pointing forwards, so that when the knees and ankles are asked to bend they bend in this plane of movement. By doing this, the basic bio-mechanical patterns of the legs are reinforced, and the feet, ankles and knees learn useful and coherent actions that help us in everyday life.

We repeat patterns not to limit us in life, but as the musician practises their scales, we practise basic patterns so we can move freely in life.

We can, of course, reduce posture practice to a sequence of muscular stretches or strengthening exercises, focusing on different parts of the body. This may loosen us up a bit, but it does not inform our nervous systems in any useful way. It does not help us to understand our habits and, perhaps more importantly, it can be counter-productive and may harm us.

Yoga is a very powerful way of integrating the mind, the body and the breath, but to do so effectively we need to pay attention to how we have evolved, how we move, breathe and respond to gravity. Only then can our practice become really productive.

The postures shown in this book are just a few examples of yoga's many side bends, forward bends, back bends and twists.

I have tried to provide pure examples of each movement pattern. In life, though, we continually make movements that involve complex combinations of patterns, and as we advance our yoga practice we find more postures that involve more than one pattern.

We repeat patterns not to limit us in life, but as the musician practises their scales, we practise basic patterns so we can move freely in life

Working with fundamental patterns helps to clarify how we move. It is common to find that when one intends to twist, one actually does something else instead, or something additional. So when we practise side bends, for example, we need to note whether we are inadvertently forward bending or backward bending, just as when twisting we might also be side-bending or flexing.

If this is happening in our yoga practice, it will most certainly be happening in our lives, which can lead to awkward and clumsy movements and, ultimately discomfort or injury.

We also need to learn to distribute patterns evenly throughout our bodies. Poorly distributed forces create stresses and strains at joints, which invariably lead to pain or discomfort and an increased likelihood of layering protective patterns over causative ones. When we take this approach, yoga becomes an inquiry into the way we engage through our bodies. It helps us notice when we do unhelpful things, and, once noticed, we can we can gently set about letting them go.

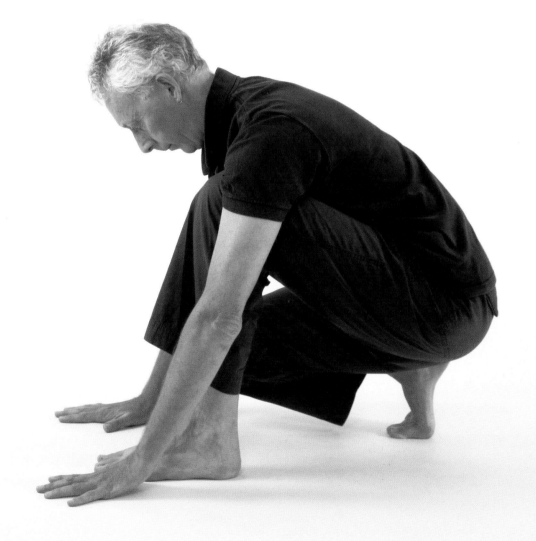

INNATE RESPONSES
OF THE BREATH TO GRAVITY
Life force and rhythm

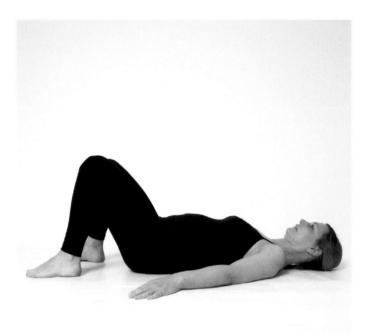

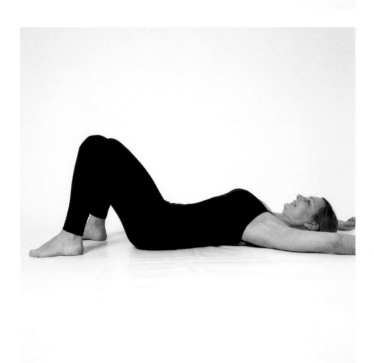

It is important to recognise the relationship between breathing and movement. When we lie on our backs with our knees bent and feet on the floor, the entire body is supported by the floor so we need no muscular response to gravity. The body will choose the easiest way to breathe, the way that involves the least effort, meaning it will always move into the softest part of the trunk.

This is nearly always the abdomen. Abdominal breathing, sometimes called diaphragmatic breathing, only requires activity in the diaphragm; the abdominal muscles themselves have to relax. The diaphragm pushes down on the contents of the abdomen and pelvis which, in turn, pushes up on the belly and down on the pelvic floor. When the diaphragm relaxes as we exhale, it moves back into the thorax and the abdominal and pelvic contents follow. The belly falls and the pelvic floor moves up. This is the natural and easy rhythm of the supine breath.

When we breathe into the chest in this supine position we move away from the natural response to a conscious one, which can be a useful enquiry. We soon find out if there is any resistance to breathing here .

While most people will find abdominal breathing easier in this position, chest breathing should not feel difficult. If we alternate between taking a belly breath and a chest breath a few times, we soon get a sense of the type of breathing we've habituated.

For chest breathers, it can be useful to lie with one hand on the belly and the other on the ribs, and to practise quiet breathing, allowing only the belly to move.

If, for example, you cannot breathe into the chest without the belly moving, then it can be helpful to practise chest breathing with the arms over the head. When we do this, the

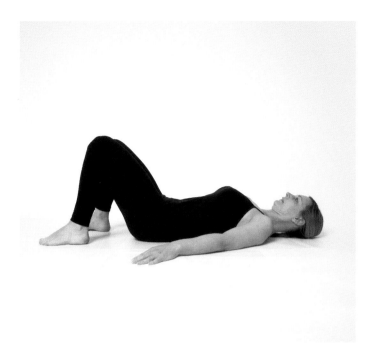

muscles running from the arms and shoulders to the ribs and lower back help to elevate the ribs mechanically, this encourages the breath to move more into the thorax and less into the belly.

In fact, in every posture where the arms are elevated, the breath will tend to move more towards the ribs and less in the belly.

It is interesting to note that when we come on to all fours, there is a natural tendency to tighten the abdominal muscles and in so doing unconsciously prevent the spine from collapsing. Again this is a reflex change, the body's response to gravity, which again impacts on breathing.

These reflex changes are a sign of well-integrated breathing and will tend to occur when unnecessary effort is reduced to a minimum.

To lose unnecessary tension we need to find adequate support from our bones. Bones are the only structural parts of the body that can transmit forces; they are, therefore, the means by which the weight of the body is transmitted to the floor.

When we allow this to happen, without tightening muscles unnecessarily, we need to become well grounded. A well-grounded body can become still, much in the way a bowl of water becomes still, if undisturbed. This is quite different to becoming stiff like a brick wall. Both may be unmoving, but only the bowl of water has the potential for movement.

When well-grounded we may be still, but the slightest impulse could initiate movement. Any unhelpful muscle tension will stiffen us and take the potential for movement away. In well-grounded movements, breathing can adjust appropriately, whereas stiffness tends to "fix" breathing.

Many of the techniques developed in yoga are designed to bring equilibrium back to the

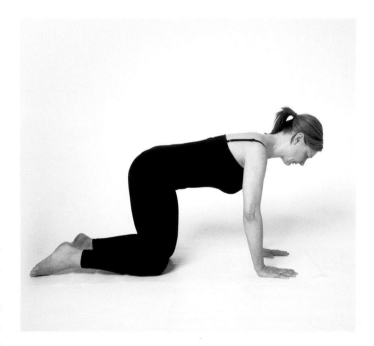

respiratory system. While the postures can help strengthen and lengthen the muscles supporting respiration, some muscles are more difficult to get to than others. These include the diaphragm, the pelvic floor and the transverse abdominus: the respiratory muscles that support the fluid core of the body.

It is here, therefore, that a more specialised approach is required, namely a mixture of breathing practices and bandha work (control of the respiratory muscles), together with some kriyas (cleansing techniques).

Innate responses of the breath to gravity – Life force and rhythm

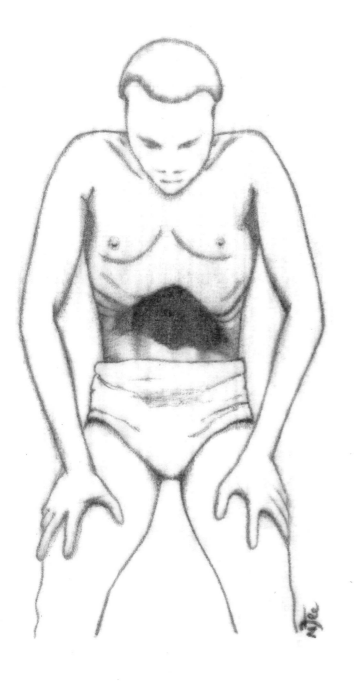

Uddiyana bandha

Uddiyana bandha is a very important practice in yoga. As far as I am aware it is the only way of consciously stretching the diaphragm.

The rib cage expands while emptied of air, creating a partial vacuum in the chest cavity. The diaphragm and everything below gets sucked upwards, stretching the diaphragm into a higher dome than it assumes during resting exhalation.

To prepare the body for this posture, one needs to be able to experience the respiratory system doing unfamiliar things. Although Uddiyana bandha is something children naturally experiment with, a lot of people lose the capacity to do it as they get older.

The following breathing exercises are very useful ways of preparing the body for this pose. They should be taken slowly and thoughtfully.

Although Uddiyana is something children naturally experiment with, a lot of people lose the capacity to do it as they get older

Step by step

1 Lying on your back with the knees bent and the feet on the floor, breathe into the belly and keep the rib cage quiet and undisturbed. This contracts the diaphragm while relaxing the belly.

2 Breathe into the chest and keep the belly quiet. This activates the rib elevator muscles, with less activity in the diaphragm.

3 Alternate between the two exercises above: one breath into the belly the next one into the chest.

4 Now try and make the belly-breath movement without breathing; expanding the belly while not actually breathing in. This is a voluntary contraction of the diaphragm with inhibition of the rib elevator muscles.

5 Try the same with the chest breath. Expand the rib cage but do not actually breathe in. This is voluntary contraction of the rib elevator muscles that inhibits the activation of the diaphragm.

6 Exhale fully and pause the breath at the end of the exhalation. Note the tension that builds up in the abdominal muscles when you exhale fully, acknowledging how the abdominals act as accessory muscles for deep exhalation by pulling the ribs together.

7 Now see if you can exhale fully and relax the abdominal muscles while the breath is held at the end of the out breath. To do Uddiyana bandha successfully, the breath needs to be fully out, but the abdominals must be relaxed.

8 Now do all the steps to stage 7, and with the breath still paused, expand the rib cage

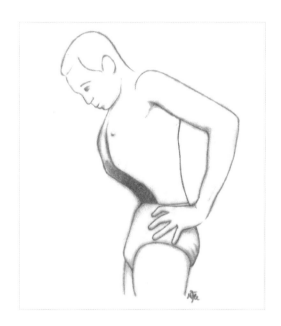

as you did in stage 5. Your abdomen will feel drawn in, because the expanded rib cage will have lowered the pressure inside the thoracic cavity and the diaphragm will be drawn up into it. The abdominal organs, abdominal wall and the pelvic floor will all move up as well. You are now doing Uddiyana bandha. It can be helpful to practise this with the arms on the floor above the head, as this helps elevate the ribs. Not only does Uddyana bandha stretch a tight diaphragm, it also draws up abdominal organs and takes pressure off the pelvic floor; both of which are compromised by a low diaphragm.

A note of caution: There are some contra-indications for Uddiyana bandha, namely inflammatory conditions of the gut including diverticulitis, Chron's disease and ulcerative colitis. Conditions such as IBS may improve with gentle Uddiyana work, as may many other digestive disorders. It is obviously inadvisable to practise this during pregnancy, or if it causes discomfort during menstruation.

Innate responses of the breath to gravity – Life force and rhythm

Kapalabhati

This breathing exercise or *kriya* is described differently in different books. Here, I describe the technique where the exhalation is the active part of the breath and the inhalation is passive. It has some useful and beneficial effects, which I'll explore as the technique is described.

Step by step

1 Sit in a comfortable position and place your finger tips about halfway between the navel and the pubic bone.

2 Imagine you are going to blow out a candle flame with one short, sharp breath. Feel what your abdominal muscles do. They should move in. A few people will find that the muscles move out instead, which is a very inefficient way of expelling air. The main muscle that should contract here is the transverse abdominal. It squeezes in, forcing the contents of the abdomen to move up against the diaphragm, which in turn pushes on the lungs from below and forces air out of them. This movement activates the transverse abdominal muscle and relaxes the diaphragm; the opposite of what so often happens in daily life, where a tense diaphragm pushes down on weakened abdominal muscles.

3 Practise blowing out your imagined candle five to 10 times with a second's pause between each one. Each time with a sharp inward contraction of the abdomen. The in breath comes in passively if you relax the abdomen between each exhalation. With practise, you should be able to blow out many times without running out of breath.

4 When you can do at least 20 exhalations comfortably, repeat the process but breathe out through the nose instead. This is Kapalabhati. If the idea of blowing out a candle does not work, you can try making a "ha" sound, which will produce a similar response in the abdomen. Although not traditionally taught this way, I tend to encourage people, especially women, to practise Kapalabhati with concomitant contraction of the pelvic floor. When the abdomen is drawn in during exhalation, the abdominal contents are pushed upwards helping expel air from the lungs. However, like the toothpaste tube that is squeezed in the middle, some of the contents will also move down against the pelvic floor. This is unhelpful and may even exacerbate problems such as stress incontinence, prolapse or haemorrhoids. Do not keep the pelvic floor muscles lifted continually, rather contract and release them with the abdominal muscles. This will bring some tone to the pelvic floor as well as the abdominal muscles.

Balanced standing pose
Tadasana or mountain posture

This is the starting position for many yoga postures. There is some natural tonus in the abdominal muscles. However, it is a mistake to think that this should be artificially held.

When the abdominal muscles are held artificially, the natural response of the belly and pelvic floor are interfered with and responsive breathing is sacrificed in favour of support. This is one of the problems caused by an over concern with ideas of core stability. Support and breathing are inextricably bound to each other: An over concern with support stifles our breathing, while softening too much for the breath compromises support. If we think we have to breathe in a particular way or "hold" ourselves in a particular way, then something else is usually sacrificed.

Many of us have lost the natural relationship between support and breathing, and it is tempting to try and solve breathing issues by teaching breathing techniques. Personally, I'm not sure it is possible to solve breathing problems unless you consider how we support ourselves – whether we over support or under support. When we address these things, breathing tends to normalise.

We should look for those subtle but important shifts that happen in the breath as we move from one posture to another. It is a big mistake to go through practice with an attitude held in the belly. While it is tempting to look for quick solutions to back problems or pelvic floor problems or any other structural issues, their causes are usually complex and take time to unravel. We need patience, curiosity and attentiveness if we are to "unpick" the things we unconsciously do that cause our problems. When we manage to do so, however, the improvements are likely to be more profound and longer lasting.

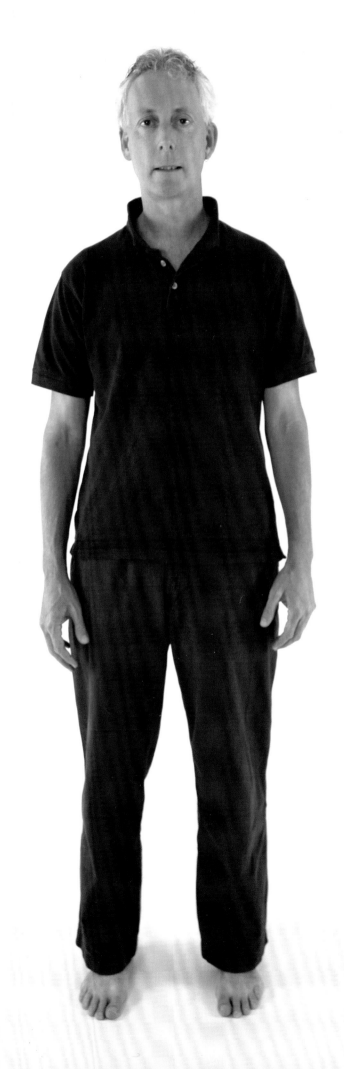

Index

172

Index

References

1   Varieties of Religious Experience, William James (Longmans, Green & Co, 1902)   **18**

2   Emotional Anatomy, Stanley Keleman (Center Press, 1985, www.centerpress.com)   **33**

3   Visceral Manipulation, Jean-Pierre Barral and Pierre J Mercier (Eastland Press, 2008)   **38**

4   Body Mechanics and Health , Leah C Thomas and Joel E Goldthwaite (Pranava Books, 2009)   **39**

5   A Basis for Sensorimotor Development - Normal and Abnormal, Mary R Fiorentino (SOS Free Stock, 1981)   **46**

6   Infant Motor Development, Jan Piek (Human Kinetics, 2005)   **47**

7   The Stress of Life, Hans Selye (McGraw-Hill, 1978)   **47**

8   Job's Body: A Handbook for Bodywork , Deane Juhan (Barrytown/Station Hill Press Inc, 2003)   **52**

9   The Yoga Tradition of the Mysore Palace, NE Sjoman (Abhinav Publications, 1999)   **56**

10   Muscles Alive: Their Functions Revealed by Electromyography, John V Basmajain and Carlo J De Luca (Williams & Wilkins, 1985)   **62**

11   Elastic Properties in Animal Movement, R McNeill Alexander (Cambridge University Press, 1988)   **64**

12   Loneliness: Human Nature and the Need for Social Connection, John T Cacioppo (WW Norton & Company, 2009)   **68**

13   Why Love Matters: How Affection Shapes a Baby's Brain, Sue Gerhardt (Routledge, 2004)   **69**

14   The Art of Loving, Eric Fromm (first published 1956)   **70**

15   Honest to God, John Robinson (SCM Press, 1963)   **70**

16   The God Delusion, Richard Dawkins (Bantam Books, 2006)   **71**

17   The Feeling of What Happens: Body and Emotion in the Making of Conciousness, Antonio Damasio (Houghton Mifflin Harcourt, 1999)   **72**

18   The Spinal Engine, Serge Gracovetsky, (Springer-Verlag, 1989)   **80**